Dementia Journey

A carer's guide to Dementia

Jennifer Muir & Blanche Antonisen

J&B Books
2023

Disclaimer
This book is memoir. The views, information or opinions expressed in *Dementia journey: A carer's guide to Dementia* are solely those of the co-authors and do not necessarily represent those of government, general practitioners, medical specialists, medical institutions, nursing homes, respite homes, or non-government institutions that provide medical support and/or information pertaining to Dementia.

ISBN 978-0-6459416-0-9 [paperback]
ISBN 978-0-6459416-1-6 [ebook]

Publisher
J&B Books
44/67 Macgregor Street, Deakin ACT 2600

Edited and designed by David Whitbread
Cover illustration from Shutterstock/Lightspring

CONTENTS

BIOGRAPHIES

Jennifer Muir OAM was born in Melbourne and attended school and university in Sydney. Jennifer travelled widely and lived in England and America where she met and later married her husband Fulton. On returning to Australia in 1981, she became a library teacher in Canberra for 15 years. She has always been committed to community service. After retiring she spent ten years as the President of a volunteer program working with primary school children, as well as balancing her commitments for a time as the National President of the Australian Women of the Year Association. When she returned to live in Canberra she and her family lived on a farm. She thoroughly enjoyed the rural life, but left to move into the leafy Canberra suburbs to be closer to her family and doctors when Fulton was diagnosed with Dementia. For two years, Jennifer cared for him in their family home prior to him moving into a nursing home, where he died a few months later. She was married to Fulton for 40 years before he passed away from Dementia in 2013. She has four children and three stepchildren. Jennifer enjoys being a proud grandmother of five. Her main interests at present include studying Latin, reading, movies and music. Jennifer has a keen sense of humour which helped her through the Dementia journey.

James Fulton Muir AO was born and educated in Melbourne. He worked as a banker in Australia, New Zealand and England before being seconded by the NSW Government to be the NSW Government Commissioner for North America. He met and married Jennifer in America and spent a number of years working there. After returning to Australia, he lived in Canberra with Jenny and their children. After his return to Canberra, he was appointed head of Westpac Bank, then Chair of the Canberra Development Board, and later Chair of the Finance Committee at the Australian National University (ANU). He received an honorary doctorate from the ANU, where the enterprise building is named in his honour for his work in commercialising the university's research. Fulton worked for many business and arts organisations, becoming president and later a life member of the Capital Arts Patrons Organisation, which supports the region's artists. He also applied his skills to Canberra-based and national organisations including the Australian Academy of Science, the CSIRO, the Australian Institute of Sport and Canberra Girls Grammar School. For his contribution to the Australian banking and community sectors, he received recognition from the Australian Government by being awarded an Order of Australia. After retiring, he enjoyed spending his weekends on his farm, fitting in a regular weekly game of golf.

Blanche Antonisen was born in Goa, a Portuguese colony until 1968, situated on the southwestern coast of India. She moved from Goa to start her school as a boarder in Karachi, Pakistan. Blanche was a boarder from age 5 to 18 at a Catholic school run by the Franciscan Missionaries of Mary until she finished school. In 1971 when the India/Pakistan war started, she had to leave Pakistan. With a Portuguese passport and unable to stay in Pakistan, a nun who had taught her now lived in Australia and recognised her refugee status and stepped in. Blanche became an Australian citizen in 1973. She married Jack Antonisen, a Dutchman she met whilst travelling. They have two daughters and four grandchildren. Blanche completed her tertiary education as an adult in Australia, gaining her Bachelor of Arts in Communication from the University of Western Sydney. A proud stay-at-home mother for 20 years, when her children were at senior school, Blanche gained employment in public relations, technical writing, and administration. She has been an active member of the community, volunteering at schools and helping people in her local community and neighbourhood. After 46 years together, with his Dementia diagnosis, Jack changed and became a stranger and Blanche took on the role of a carer 24/7. After Jack died, Blanche spent 18 months overseas, learning creative writing in New York, and renting an apartment in London to get to know her English grandkids and travel around Europe. Blanche enjoys reading, belongs to a book club, appreciates the arts, takes nature and healthy cooking seriously, and her regular travels have enhanced her cultural sensitivity, to adopt and adapt to globalisation and its benefits.

Jack Antonisen was born in the Netherlands and completed his secondary, tertiary and professional education in Holland. He was employed by an international firm of chartered accountants. His career lent itself to travel, helped by his being fluent in four languages. On completing his professional education at 22, Jack left Holland for England and worked in London, Rotterdam, Paris, New York, Singapore and Sydney. He enjoyed the opportunity to immerse himself in the culture, politics, art, classical music, gardening and nature whilst working. After accumulating both cash and work experience, his zest to see the world kicked in again. Jack decided to put accounting to one side and threw himself into travel for five years. He sold his French sports car, bought a guitar and took a train from Paris to Iran, and then a boat to the Far East. He spent years travelling through the Middle East, India, Central America, the US, Canada, Australia and New Zealand, and returned home to Europe in the autumn of 1972. He decided to return to Australia where he had a job waiting and to marry Blanche. When their two children left home, Blanche and Jack travelled extensively around the world but, sadly it all came to a halt when Jack was diagnosed with Dementia with Lewy Bodies in 2011. A man who so valued stability and predictability in life, Jack struggled to understand why he had been afflicted with this disease and tried to figure out how he could 'beat it'. But no amount of intellect, exercise or medication could help overcome his frustration. This became his ongoing battle to the end. However, his final weeks and days were dignified and peaceful, as he no longer fought it. Instead, he directed the same energy to connect as best he could with his wife, his two daughters and their husbands, and his four grandchildren, to the very end.

How it all began

Hi Jenny

I understand from our friend Ellnor, who's more like a family member than a friend, that she has already been in touch with you about Jack's recent Lewy Body Dementia (LBD) diagnosis, and she has given me your email address so I can call on you for help.

Ellnor informs me that you are the best person to turn to for help, as you've had several years of experience caring for your husband Fulton at your home.

What a coincidence that both Jack and Fulton have been diagnosed with the same type of Dementia.

Jenny, I wish to share so much with you and welcome your input and hope this long email is not overwhelming.

I understand from Ellnor you're now in the process of finding a nursing home for Fulton, as his care needs have reached a point where it's no longer safe to care for him at home. I wish you luck in finding a nursing home soon, and hopefully it won't be as big a challenge as an early diagnosis has been for us.

In all the years I've known Ellnor, I've never known her to decline to help anyone with a simple 'no', and she actually admitted she has no idea how to help! I can understand her fear as I'm also fearful with the little encouragement, knowledge and support I receive from my Dementia courses that I enrolled in for the next six weeks.

Jack and I have already attended a few Dementia workshops and there's much emphasis on establishing a good daily routine from the start. Jack and I would both benefit from a daily routine and it will give us predictability in our otherwise chaotic world.

I am making every effort to learn and understand the disease with the classes Jack and I attended, these courses run by Dementia Australia. The staff are ever ready with their encouragement and information. We were told they're there to help and guide carers to the excellent resources that are available in the community. Sadly, the access to these resources only becomes available once the diagnosis is delivered. I have been given several options that I have yet to follow.

The workshop I attended last week informed all carers to start the nursing home search now and not to leave it until it's too late!

Now that I am living in a Dementia world, I often find myself searching for blogs where people who have recently been diagnosed write about their illness and they narrate their stories vividly, how they cope with their on-going loss, and living in isolation sometimes helps to understand the disease.

In one of my readings, I learnt that although many people worldwide are affected with Dementia, yet carers still start their journey in a silent world, confused and unable to make sense of what is unfolding before their eyes and, worse still, there's little help until the Dementia is diagnosed.

When Ellnor visited our home, she noticed the high levels of stress and exhaustion that I was under. Jack is unable to share in the household duties. Worse still, I now have the added responsibility of having to watch him like a toddler.

Jenny, can you please help with any strategies that you had in place and that worked for you? A routine will work well for Jack as he was so predictable in his routine and this would bring him comfort if he knows what is expected of him each day. I have bought a whiteboard and write up our daily schedules and visits and I often find him reading these notes. This way I don't have to repeat myself, I just tell him, 'Please Jack, check the notes on the whiteboard.'

Ellnor is unaware but she unknowingly lessened my feelings of isolation and loneliness by introducing you. She telephoned to let me know that she has already spoken to you and you have agreed to help when I am ready.

I cannot stress how fortunate I feel to get help from another carer, as this makes me feel connected, not only to you but your real lived stories, and to understand the disease through your lived experiences. No book or research information can be as ready a guide as you are.

I am also well aware that I cannot expect to have the same experiences as you had with Fulton, because the process of the disease is played out differently for each person.

It has been brought to my notice that depression symptoms can sometimes mimic Dementia symptoms. Jack has suffered with mild depression symptoms for years, but it was brought under control with prescription medication.

Ellnor tells me that you struggled enormously in caring for Fulton in the early days, with no training and you had to learn by trial and error. Even when Fulton's needs became high-care you were unaware of where to seek help and had even less idea of what were the important questions that needed to be addressed with the medical staff.

Jenny, can you cope with re-living Fulton's early stages of Dementia to assist me?

Even though I know Ellnor very well and see her frequently, I am uncomfortable in discussing Jack's delusional attacks. Nor can I bring myself to have the conversation with our children. Our youngest daughter Maria is a Registered Nurse, but is now tied up with a young family and has enough on her plate. I also have another daughter who lives in London who is unable to help due to the distance. Besides I don't want to talk about Jack's personality changes with our girls, as I wish to keep their memories of him intact.

Jenny, many thanks in advance, for taking the time to hear me out today.

I know there is a team of resourceful people out there who want to change the attitudes to how Dementia is viewed, but I'm uncomfortable to speak to strangers about our personal life.

Jenny, thanks again for all your help and support and it is greatly appreciated.

Kind regards

Blanche

***

Dear Blanche

Ellnor had mentioned you may contact me regarding your husband's diagnosis with Dementia.

My husband Fulton also has Dementia with Lewy Bodies, so they will have a lot of similar behaviours. As a result, I completely understand what you are going through. The disease is so challenging and sad.

I am only too happy to provide you with whatever assistance and support I can to help you in your caring role. As Jack is still living at home, you will have a number of decisions to make regarding his future care. I felt quite guilty about deciding I could no longer care for Fulton at home, but it became impossible for me to function with no sleep and his increasingly challenging behaviours.

Fulton was diagnosed only two years ago, and he remained at home until about September this year.

He is now in the final stage of Dementia and is totally calm and peaceful. Sadly, he has been confined to an invalid chair since returning from hospital after a bout of pneumonia, as he cannot walk. However, I'm pleased that he is no longer fighting his illness but is comfortable and is well cared for by the nursing home staff.

I visit him daily just because I want to be with him but also to make sure he is being well cared for by the staff. I have heard terrible stories about maltreatment of the patients in nursing homes, but I have found no evidence of this where he is. I do think it is a good idea to arrive and leave at irregular times, this way I can meet all the staff working on different shifts.

Every day is emotionally draining as I don't know if he will be here tomorrow. Fulton is serene and calm, as for him the battle is over.

I vowed to myself that when Fulton passed away I would try to help anyone on this journey in any way I could.

It is quite serendipitous that you approached me for help just when our journey is coming to an end. Sometimes, all you may need is for someone to listen. I know I have not wanted to share some of my problems with the children, especially those relating to our relationship, as I don't feel it would be appropriate, and I feel for them as they have their own grief to handle.

Fulton was a very private person and so I have tried to preserve his dignity by not sharing all his confronting behaviours with our children. Yes, it is hard to no longer have a loving relationship or even a relationship at all with your husband on this Dementia journey.

So I am happy about trying to help you on your Dementia journey as it may help me to heal.

I told Ellnor I would help you if I possibly could. I am conscious though that I do not have all the answers. I too believe that unless you have been on this Dementia caring journey you cannot begin to understand how emotionally draining and physically challenging it can be.

Continue to reach out to others through the Alzheimer's Association as you may find answers to some of your issues.

I look forward to hearing from you anytime you need a listener.

Good luck with the ACAT team [Aged Care Assessment Team], I found them to be most sympathetic and understanding.

Kind regards

Jenny

***

Hi Jenny

Jenny you've no idea what a great support and strength you are, having made yourself readily available to provide assistance. I find I am no longer guessing or muddling on my own, as I can count on you to make sense of the confusing nature of the disease as it unfolds. One minute Jack appears normal and in a flash I can have a behavioural episode.

Jenny, you give me great comfort with our daily chats and with our regular email exchanges.

You talk honestly and plainly of your journey with Fulton. You have warned me that the Dementia experience for Jack will be different from Fulton's, especially as Jack also has Parkinson's. You correctly point out that these were two separate Dementias and will affect his cognition and his physicality.

Jenny, before you arrived on the scene as a listening post and support, I felt confused and unable to navigate through this Dementia maze. You've no idea how your level of support to listen and have the level of conversation that provided me with examples of Fulton's episodes, has changed my perspective immediately. I learnt it was best to just observe and care, and not to try and make sense of the disease. You've made me aware that it's the only 'correct way' to act, as there is little I can do to change the situation and there will come a time when the disease will slowly grip and destroy Jack's brain noticeably and the challenging behaviours will only manifest more frequently.

I appreciate you giving me the gift of empowerment that makes the daily grind of understanding Dementia easier. Your support has allowed me to manage this complex disease.

I've taken on board your advice and have now established the first step of creating a good reliable routine, which helps me immensely as a carer. The daily routine in place now brings some predictability in our otherwise chaotic world.

You will be interested to hear that the Alzheimer's conference I attended in Sydney was well attended and it has left me a little empowered to know there's plenty of help and support around for carers. Better still, a woman approached me who was a past carer and gave me details for a nursing home in the vicinity, where I plan to buy my new home. I'll check the nursing home as the recommendations are beyond belief!

Soon I'll have the added stress as I will have to prepare our home for sale and it's indeed daunting to even think of the four decades of possessions I'll have to declutter. The house has to go for sale, so I've the finances to pay the nursing home bond.

Thanks again for your time and support.
It's indeed very appreciated.
Blanche

***

Dear Blanche
You too have gone through a frustrating path to Jack's diagnosis with Dementia, but for totally different reasons than I did with Fulton.

Fulton was not exactly a model patient. He hated going to a doctor and I think had only consulted a doctor a couple of times during our marriage. The first time was for a hernia operation, the second was a knee operation and the third was when prostate cancer was diagnosed.

Sadly, when the Dementia diagnosis was made, he had reached the final stage of the disease. It was then really too late for medication to help him. By then he was fearful of strangers. I could only leave him at home with one of the children. This restricted my ability to leave our home, except in his company. So I could not attend any of the Alzheimer's Association meetings. Nor would he attend respite day care. A late diagnosis makes everything so much harder for the carer and the family.

A doctor told me recently that Dementia is difficult to diagnose and that often doctors prefer to test for everything else they think their patient may have, before testing for Dementia. When I asked her why this was so, she said there is so much stigma with such a diagnosis that it changes how a patient feels about everything. So she felt it better to delay diagnosis as long as possible. Maybe that is why only when Jack and Fulton became advanced in their Dementia journey a definitive diagnosis was confirmed.

At least now it is easier for me to cope, as I know Fulton could not control his behaviour any more than a two-year-old child can.

A dear friend of ours is flying over from Perth for a final visit with Fulton tomorrow. These goodbyes are so sad and I hate coming home to my empty house afterwards to sit alone with my memories.

Loneliness and isolation are the two feelings that are faced by us carers on a daily basis.

Think tonight I need a 'cheer up' phone call!

Love
Jenny

***

Dear Jenny
Jenny, you're an absolutely a godsend.

I'm unable to talk to the children about my stress level that everyday caring for their father brings. Jack often doesn't cooperate because he hasn't given up and still likes to understand his day-to-day care. Besides I can understand the children want to remember him as their 'super' dad!

I often ask myself if I ever will get over the LBD diagnosis? I'm now almost totally obsessed with all things Dementia and find myself wanting to talk, read, write and research answers to this horrible and devastating diagnosis.

Jenny, I want you to know that most of my answers comes from the information you have shared about your caring journey with Fulton. You have the ability to explain this complex disease in clear plain English!

You also bring me hope and strength, by telling me to take each day as it comes. But then you confuse me further, by warning me that no day is the same!

Thanks for also bringing to my notice that Dementia stages do not unfold in a linear pattern, that one morning I'll wake up and find Jack displaying middle stages of his Dementia, and later on the same day he's back to stage one. The message I receive from you is, 'do your best' as the circumstances arise. In one of my readings, I learnt that the brain is a delicate and complicated instrument that once faulty is difficult to put right!

Before the Dementia diagnosis, Jack had a brilliant mind and now it's foggy and in recent times I find this most unfortunate as I don't recognise the man I'm living with. Gone is the articulate communicator, now replaced by a man who's hesitant and his conversation often makes little sense.

To get any action or response, I find I have to encourage and motivate him. This constant encouragement is now always one way only and draining!

The equality in our relationship is now gone, and a stranger has moved in, and this stranger is unable to share in the household tasks. For that matter, he is even unable to care for himself independently. I lay out his clothes each morning and he can no longer manage the buttons on his shirt. Now that I am thinking for two people, there are times my brain, due to sheer exhaustion, is unable to think rationally and sometimes I find myself acting on impulse when a quick decision has to be made, and wonder if I too am getting Dementia.

There are times too when I feel I'm losing control and patience as Jack digs his heels in. This is when I practise mindfulness, taking slow calculated breaths. Jenny, the wise words you bring into our nightly conversation, are slowly coming home to roost, yet LBD can still bring its own share of new challenges. There are days I get it so wrong and want to run away. But with your help I'm getting resilient as a carer.

I have noticed our family dynamics are no longer the same. Nor can the family function the way it did in the past, as it is now fractured with the girls unable to take equal responsibility for the care of their father. Although I keep both girls informed about Jack's up-to-date care plans. To me this information is crucial, as this way they can make plans to visit their father.

Naturally, I am heartbroken how our children are drifting, and I am unable to raise my concerns with Jack. All I can do at the moment is to be realistic and not foster competition among them.

Luckily, I am not old and in relatively good health, to manage Jack's care on my own, without engaging their assistance, time, support or even to rely on their financial assistance.

Again, thank you for giving me your time, until next time.

Kind regards

Blanche

***

Hi Blanche

It was good to chat last night. Sometimes I, like you, have had a 'shocker of a day'. Then a coffee with a friend or a late-night chat on the phone may be just the stress relief I need. So I'm glad I was able to help you. It is so hard to explain to family and friends the multiplicity of Dementia-related issues you and I have to handle every day. So talking to someone who has been on the journey and understands what you are going through can lighten your load somewhat.

I remember one night not long after the diagnosis I woke up and found Fulton fully dressed in his business suit standing in our dressing room. I tried to speak calmly, although I was really worried. 'Darling, you don't go to work anymore. Remember? You retired a year ago.'

He looked at me quizzically, 'Don't tell me you have forgotten my finance meeting? I am the Chair so it's imperative I go to the office early to prepare my report. I need you to drive me or I will have to call a taxi?'

My mind raced, what should I say, what can I do? It was 3am, hardly an appropriate time to go to his office. It was no good reasoning with Fulton that it was the middle of the night and he had retired from work a year ago; his mind was playing tricks with him. So I said, 'It's a bit early to go yet, I'll make coffee and we can wait awhile.'

Thankfully I had chosen the right approach as he calmly grabbed his briefcase and we went downstairs to the kitchen. I turned on Fulton's favourite movie – Lawrence of Arabia *– which fortunately lasts for almost three hours. He sat on the sofa shuffling through his papers but soon he became engrossed in the movie and fell asleep. I crept upstairs and changed from my pyjamas into my clothes, then went downstairs to wait with Fulton for the morning carer. I sat reading till the doorbell went around 7:30.*

The carer looked surprised to find Fulton full dressed in a suit. She remarked, 'You've been up early?'

Fulton replied, 'Yes, I had a very important early meeting.'

She smiled knowingly and said to Fulton, 'Let's go and change into casual clothes for your golf club lunch meeting today.'

Another potential disaster had been averted by going along with Fulton's Dementia hallucinations!

Earlier on our journey if this had happened, I would have tried to reason with Fulton, but I have found that can lead to tantrums. As you perhaps have already discovered, caring for a person who has Dementia is all trial and error. I soon found out to go along with Fulton and not argue. You too will make mistakes, but being a carer is all trial and error.

Thank you for those kind words in your last email, I am so pleased my advice helps you.

I have been quite traumatised by my journey as Fulton's carer, as so many tasks and experiences I have had to complete were totally outside my range of life knowledge and my comfort zone. Initially I could not believe what was involved, not just for Fulton but for me as his carer. I vowed to myself that when I was free, then I would try to help others placed in this invidious position. Now I know what post-traumatic stress means!

Corresponding with you is helping me to heal, not from the grief of slowly losing my husband but from the whole two years of this traumatic Dementia journey.

Every morning Fulton would look at our white board and say, 'What are we doing today?' Having a visible diary was useful for the carers too as they could see what we had on that day. Sadly, once he could no longer read, it was useless for him, but I have kept it in my pantry as a sad reminder of my life living with Dementia.

I will call you tonight to see how you went with visits to the nursing homes and how you now feel after them.
Cheers
Jenny

***

Dear Blanche
Now Fulton has died I have had time to myself for the first time in years. Time to rest and to think about my caring role with Fulton.

I was so lost when Fulton was diagnosed with Dementia.

I had no idea what Dementia was. Nor did I have any idea what caring duties would involve.

Now I am more determined than ever to write about the whole journey I have been on, to help other carers to learn and what to expect.

A number of other carers like yourself have sought me out to help them through their own Dementia caring role. I am happy to advocate for them, but I really feel the need to write down what I have learned.

I know you feel the same way, so in the future let's get together and have a chat about the way forward.

***

A year later when Jack died, Blanche travelled overseas and spent 18 months with her daughter, friends and relatives in the USA, London and Europe, and then returned to Australia revived!

We had already discussed our intention to collaboratively write our stories long before. Blanche embarked on this long trip and on her return, she started writing her part of the Dementia experiences ...

Chapter 1

Diagnosis journey

Early warning symptoms

❧

JENNY AND FULTON'S STORY

Dear Blanche

If only we knew then what we know now about Dementia, what a difference that knowledge would have made to our roles as carers.

Sharing our stories, supporting each other during those difficult days has been invaluable.

So many wasted years not knowing what was wrong with Fulton, but that all changed when we received his diagnosis ...

***

Recently I was watching a documentary on the 2004 Tsunami which engulfed the beautiful tourist beaches in Bali. I was momentarily moved by the beauty and tranquillity of the scenery and understood why the tourists were momentarily mesmerised by the scene which unfolded before them. They had no comprehension of what the receding ocean signified. Nor did they know that the huge wave, which was visible on the horizon, was a tsunami slowly moving towards the beach.

But some of the local people did know what was about to happen from their shared community knowledge of the ocean learned from past tsunamis. Shouts of 'Tsunami coming' echoed around some of the beachside resorts.

The documentary revealed many local people knew the signs of impending catastrophe and ran towards the hills when they saw the ocean receding. Even the elephants which ambled along the beach tracks carrying tourists suddenly took off for the hills.

However, many unsuspecting tourists continued to walk down on the beach to inspect the unusual phenomena of an ocean free beach. All the signs were there, signifying a tsunami was imminent, but unless you knew what the signs signified there was no way of comprehending what lay ahead.

We did not recognise the signs of Dementia that Fulton had exhibited in the years leading up to his Dementia diagnosis.

I empathised with those tourists, as I did not recognise all the symptoms Fulton displayed signified he had Dementia. Neither of us knew what ahead of us when finally we did learn of his Dementia diagnosis. We did however experience the devastation to our lives which our own Dementia tsunami caused.

I wish I could tell you that diagnosing Dementia is relatively easy. But unfortunately I found the journey to diagnosis to be long, confusing and eventually heartbreaking. To make things more challenging there are numerous types of Dementia having a multitude of symptoms and there is no cure.

Diagnosing Dementia is unlike diagnosing most other medical diseases, disorders or conditions. With prostate or breast cancer for example, a blood test, biopsy or ultrasound may provide sufficient information to reach a diagnosis relatively quickly. These procedures may be done easily and the whole process may only take a week.

This rather predictable path to diagnosis does not usually occur when diagnosing Dementia during the onset of the disease when cognitive impairment may not be obvious.

A person with Dementia may exhibit many symptoms which can mask its presence – such as depression, anxiety, confusion, mood swings, hearing loss, or memory impairment, to name a few. It is therefore possible for the consulting doctor to miss Dementia being the main physiological cause of these medical conditions.

Certainly, I had many indications over a number of years that something was amiss with Fulton.

Blanche and Jack experienced a similar change in Jack's physical and mental 'wellbeing' prior to his diagnosis. However that is where the similarities between the two men's Dementia diagnoses ended.

As with everything else involving Dementia, the age, personality, lifestyle and career of the individual has a significant impact on how and when a Dementia diagnosis is reached. Nothing is straightforward.

However an MRI will likely show the plaque growing on the brain which is a major indicator of Dementia. Sadly, by the time Fulton's doctor requested this test, Fulton's Dementia had progressed into the advanced stage.

So although Jack and Fulton both had Dementia with Lewy Bodies, our journeys to their diagnoses were totally different.

Blanche and I did however share the similar rollercoaster ride which all partner carers experience, both before and after, obtaining a definitive diagnosis. It was an extremely difficult and lonely time for us both until we unexpectedly met. Then for the first time we could share the burden of caring for a person having Dementia with somebody experiencing a similar journey. Unless you have walked in our footsteps, you would not have any idea of the physical and emotional commitment and toll caring takes in every aspect of your life.

As you may be aware, there are many different kinds of Dementia that affect people in a multitude of ways. Each individual Dementia journey is unique, as is the length of time it may take your doctor to confirm a Dementia diagnosis. Also we found the treatments suggested by our doctors varied markedly, despite our husbands both being diagnosed with Lewy Body Dementia. Some diagnoses may take months and involve a multitude of tests and procedures as Jack's did. Others like Fulton's may be one definitive test when he already was so advanced into the disease that very little could be done for him medically to help alleviate the effect of Dementia on his body.

If you are not familiar with how a person changes when Dementia is diagnosed, I advise you to read the 'Help notes' from the Alzheimers Association of NSW. It lists the stages through which the disease transitions and the accompanying behavioural and physical changes that may occur. This will give you an idea of what to expect or anticipate on your journey and to learn about the behaviours which may be exhibited by a person with Dementia.

I am sure many people traverse a similar long convoluted path that Fulton and I walked in the years prior to his diagnosis with Dementia. It takes time to receive a diagnosis as it is not an easy disease to diagnose in its early stages.

There is still a real stigma in the community about having Dementia because of a lack of knowledge about the nature of the disease. This may be the reason that some doctors have a reluctance to even suggest Dementia as a possible diagnosis in the early stages. It took many years for Fulton to be diagnosed with Dementia even though he had a number of the symptoms.

This delay may be accompanied by the doctor prescribing medications for the mood swings, anxiety and depression characteristic of this early stage of Dementia. There may also be additional treatment offered such as a course of vitamin therapy for lethargy.

I believe the treatment regimes offered may be the easiest options for a doctor, but they deny time from the person having Dementia. Time to get one's affairs in order and to share precious moments with the family before cognition is totally impacted and full enjoyment of life becomes difficult.

Some of the symptoms may also appear similar to, or can be confused with, other serious health disorders and mental illness, including psychotic hallucinations.

Dementia can impact some people when they are very young, early onset Dementia, or may not be diagnosed until a person is in their eighties. It is not an inherited condition. While in its early stages it is not an easy disease to diagnose, I believe it should be considered as a possibility during the diagnostic process rather than its possible presence being ignored.

In a way it would have been easier on us both had Fulton been diagnosed with almost anything other than Dementia. His earlier diagnosis with prostate cancer was much easier to comprehend and cope with as we both already knew what this meant.

Charitable foundations collect millions of dollars each year for research into a range of these readily recognisable diseases, which raises community awareness. But little is done in this regard for people with Dementia.

Even in 2023 there really is scant knowledge about Dementia in the general community.

This is probably why I did not even suspect Fulton had Dementia when his behaviours and personality changed markedly over a number of years. I just put the changes down to his advancing age and fatigue due to working too hard.

Even now the stereotypical view of a person with Dementia is of someone who has 'lost their marbles'. Initially he certainly did not appear to have done that. There is still a real stigma about Dementia, mainly relating it to madness in a medieval way, which I found to be just unconscionable.

I think this may be a contributing factor as to why our doctors hesitated in diagnosing Dementia, or even suggesting it as a possible diagnosis, as they believed it perhaps could be a traumatic diagnosis for the family.

Recently things have started to change, thankfully more authors are writing about Dementia now and films like *Still Alice* are providing insight into the nature of the disease for the average person. So now more people understand a little about Dementia and the impact its diagnosis may have on the whole family.

I had been in total denial in the years leading up to Fulton's diagnosis. I knew he was changing and something was wrong with him but chose to go along with his refusal to seek a medical opinion. He too must have known his cognitive ability was changing but would not admit this to anyone. He was in total denial that he could have a serious health issue. There had been a distinct change in his personality over the past five years which had manifested in depression, anxiety and mood swings.

He was a very intelligent and astute man so I believe now that masking the on-going deterioration of cognitive skills must have been relatively easy for him at first. In hindsight, I realise that keeping up the pretence of normalcy over a number of years must have caused him incredible stress.

When he was at home he developed a coping mechanism of wandering away from social gatherings to disappear into the garden, where he must have felt at ease in the calm, rural environment of our farm. At the time I could not understand why he often seemed so rude by this behaviour, to visiting friends and family. I believe now he could not follow the rapid banter of our guests and was confused by being forced to participate in conversations and social interaction in our home. I cannot imagine how difficult the university business meetings must have been for him at work.

During the years leading up to Fulton's diagnosis I too was in denial as to the severity of his illness and the impact it was having on the family. I should have insisted he consult his doctor instead of giving in to his denial of having a problem with his health. He was a very determined man and I had little chance of convincing him that his condition needed the intervention of a doctor.

At the time I had no idea he actually had an illness but believed he was starting to show signs of ageing. At no stage did any of his work colleagues express any concern about his health or his work output to me. So I decided it best not to 'rock the boat'.

When he became irrational I chose to ignore him and to hope tomorrow would be a better day. Each of the children were caught up in their own lives and I tried not to burden them with our problems. I was trying to maintain normalcy in a totally abnormal environment, hoping that the following day would not be as bad as the day before.

This was a period where due to his extreme behavioural shifts, I would try to diffuse any given situation, hoping that he would calm down. Though at the back of my mind, I would be thinking this is the quiet before the next storm.

One example of his extreme mood shifts occurred when our daughter Bianca turned 40. I invited the family home to have a small celebration including her two young children, Millie and Liam, plus our other adult children. I had been away with Alycia on one of her research trips, so Fiona had volunteered to get everything ready prior to our arrival back in Canberra. Fiona hung up decorations in our living room, so the room would look festive and set up the dining table with the birthday cake and some birthday food treats.

Fulton started to criticise everything that Fiona had done, saying the prepared food looked ridiculous and how unsuitable the decorations were for an adult's birthday. Fiona tried to reason with her father, telling him the decorations were there so the children (Millie was then eleven and Liam eight at that time) who could see it was a special celebration for their mother.

Fulton continued making sarcastic comments to us, becoming more and more agitated every minute. He was very rude and just nasty and refused to calm down. Who was this cranky old man? This was so hard for Fiona and I to cope with, especially as it was so out of character for Fulton to behave this way as he had always enjoyed our family 'get togethers' and participated in these types of celebrations with great enthusiasm. That day I dreaded the rest of the family arriving as I felt instead of being happy it would all end in tears.

However just as I thought I would have to cancel the whole thing, Fulton's mood changed quickly. It was as if the fog had lifted and he sat down and it appeared he had reverted to happy Fulton. We all relaxed for a while. The rest of the family arrived, and being unaware of what had happened prior to their arrival, no more was said about the stupid decorations.

We were able to celebrate Bianca's birthday by lighting the candles and singing 'Happy birthday' before Fulton abruptly left the room to go and watch television. I breathed a sigh of relief that yet another potential scene had been avoided.

This rollercoaster of behaviours I found so hard to adapt to as afterwards Fulton did not seem to remember what he had said or done – and it took me a long time to forgive some of these outbursts. During this phase I felt like I was walking on eggshells most of the time.

I now feel it would be best to involve your close family in the diagnostic process. Each member of the family will probably have perceived different changes in personality and behaviour and possibly have noticed memory lapses or other symptoms.

It is a difficult journey as the person with the condition may not have the cognitive ability to understand the full impact of the diagnosis or to explain what they are experiencing as they transition into Dementia.

Losing a father, mother, husband, wife, partner, grandmother or grandfather to any illness is traumatic. The burden of dealing with a terminal illness can be lightened if the family learns together and can share whatever difficulties may lie ahead. However adult children have their own lives to lead. They may not even be living nearby so often the wife or partner has to take on the journey to diagnosis alone, which is a significant part of the carers role.

Fortunately, I was not in this position as our family rallied around and helped us as much as they possibly could do.

A Dementia diagnosis may be quite traumatic and heartbreaking. But in some cases it can be a relief, as it was when Fulton was finally diagnosed by a specialist in gerontology. This was more than five years after he had first shown many symptoms of its presence. I was not Dementia aware then when these symptoms first started to appear!

After diagnosis I knew what was the cause of the many challenges which had arisen in our relationship over the past few years. The children knew at last why their father was behaving erratically and irrationally, why he was depressed and why he sometimes seemed to be unreasonably angry.

The main issues had centred around his rather unpredictable behaviours and sudden mood swings, plus he became depressed easily over the most trivial occurrence such as a missing shirt or pair of socks. This became a trigger for his paranoia which led him to believe I, or one of our adult children, was hiding things from him on purpose. During this time his mood swings were unpredictable and the whole family commented to me from time to time on some of his bizarre behaviours.

My frequent suggestions he should consult with our doctor were met with a sarcastic, 'What for?'

As he was in his seventies and still working full time in a demanding role at the university, the family put his changed personality down to the pressures of his job and advancing age.

His whole life he had been a workaholic. We all tried at different times to discuss with him the possibility of retirement but then he always became angry and confrontational. So we soon gave up on that. It was just not worth the days of anger or the nervous laughter and sarcastic commentary which followed after one of our chats about retirement.

He refused to rest. So after a busy week at work he threw himself into a frenetic weekend of farm chores like moving the cattle to a different paddock, mending fences, priming the pump or filling holes along our private road.

I could see a humorous side to all this and sometimes felt I was living on a Monty Python film set! I found it best not to question why he was doing certain things repetitively. I felt if he was happy that was all that mattered.

During one of these periods of frenzied physical work I noticed he seemed to be doing some tasks over and over again each weekend unnecessarily. I think he moved our pot plants from one side of the verandah to the other at least twenty times.

At the back of my mind I knew it was my duty to keep trying to encourage him to retire and seek medical help. But how would I achieve these goals?

I saw an opportunity one afternoon when Fulton appeared to be calmer than usual and agreed to stop working for a break from his chores. Fiona saw us both sitting outside on the verandah, she came and joined us for a chat then disappeared inside, appearing shortly afterwards with a platter of cheeses and nibbles and poured us both a glass of red wine. Soon afterwards she disappeared inside, leaving Fulton and I sitting in the sun enjoying the beautiful view out over our pool and garden to the surrounding hills. Our cattle were in the paddock nearby and a few kangaroos were grazing contentedly.

It was a perfect setting in which to relax contentedly and discuss our future plans.

We sat and talked for a long time about finally retiring and travelling in Europe. Fulton seemed to be relaxed and was engaged in our conversation. I was heartened by this. Maybe at last he might agree to travel and start the holiday we had planned for years.

However, no luck, he suddenly stood up abruptly and said, 'You live in "la-la-land". I have to work for a few more years to finish what needs to be done at the university. The farm does not run itself – and I have absolutely no interest in travelling any more.'

He called out to Fiona to, 'Come here, I have something to tell you. Fiona, why don't you take your mother on a European cruise? She's been planning to do that for years. She obviously needs a holiday!'

(Of course, Fiona had no interest in doing that as she had her own plans.)

He continued, 'Now, thanks for the snack, but I have to return to fixing the road. I have too much work to do. I just have not got the time left to waste on holidays. But I am happy for you two to go whenever you like.'

Hardly the response I wanted to hear! Then he left to return to work on our road, yet again.

Thus, despite the hopeful beginning, yet another effort to discuss retirement was derailed by Fulton refusing to confront reality. This was repeated many times over the next few years. All our children tried in different ways to convince him that it was time to stop working full time. However nobody had any success at all. In fact, as time went by he became more determined to stay working.

But why was he so fixated on maintaining the status quo? It was only after he was diagnosed with Dementia that I received a satisfactory answer to this question.

So I found the years leading up to Fulton's diagnosis incredibly challenging for this and many other reasons. It was sad as we had planned to go and live overseas for a year while we revisited and explored our favourite cities and countries. Added to his refusal to consider retirement were his daily frustrations with his inability to carry on with life as it used to be.

I was annoyed by his refusal to seek medical advice and especially annoyed by his refusal to at least cut back on his work hours at the university.

He kept losing things like his keys to his car or to his university office, causing problems for all of us who were trying to help him. He had often lost things in the past, but what changed now was he would blame anyone around for hiding whatever was missing.

He often complained to me that his staff kept changing things on his computer but he refused to ask them to help him. Rather he requested one of us, either Alycia or Fiona, should go into his office with him at the weekend to help him do previously easy things like accessing and sending emails. He told us the technical staff were changing the software on his computer and he kept forgetting his password on his home and office computers. He became totally confused by anything to do with his computer, yet he had been computer literate and had used one for years. Sadly, during our visits to his office we could see that he could no longer compose or even send an email without great difficulty.

Being invited to write a speech propelled him into days of suppressed rage and overt anxiety, even though it was acknowledged that he was an excellent public speaker in the past. For many years he had been invited to make speeches for a range of business, school and community groups. He took great pleasure in doing this and enjoyed the accolades he received. It was something he took great pleasure in doing. Now he resented being asked to give a speech. Our individual efforts to help him prepare a speech only caused him to become agitated and annoyed.

We were damned if we helped him – and damned if we did not.

I believe this constant see-sawing of emotions and behaviours indicated that something could be dreadfully wrong with him physically. He catastrophised the most trivial issue.

For some time I thought he was becoming senile but then I began to think perhaps he had a brain tumour. However, as usual he ignored my repeated requests for him to seek medical attention in order to gain a diagnosis for his ever-increasing odd behaviour.

But just as I was despairing about him and wondering what to do next, he would bounce back to his former happy-go-lucky disposition. It was as if a mist had cleared and he could see things more clearly. Then he would again fall into a fog of despondency. The whole family went on this rollercoaster ride with Fulton. It only worsened as time went by.

In hindsight, this change in disposition and unpredictable behaviours appear to be characteristic of people having

Dementia. This can put many relationships under pressure during those months or years prior to a definitive diagnosis. It is possible that some breakdowns in long-term family relationships and marriages could be attributed to undiagnosed Dementia. Fortunately, we managed to ride out this stormy period and, for a year prior to diagnosis, Fulton's previous loving happy disposition reappeared.

One Sunday we had invited some friends to join us for a swim and barbeque, something which had happened many times in the past. On this day Fulton was pouring drinks for all, but I noticed he was pouring a full glass of vodka and just topping it off with Bloody Mary mix.

I said, 'Fulton, what are you doing?'

He replied sarcastically, 'Getting drinks for everyone – what does it look like?'

I was shocked at his rudeness in front of our friends, and by his confrontational tone. He slammed the vodka bottle down and stormed off outside and did not join us again that afternoon. He disappeared to work on yet another 'project'. He stayed outside for the rest of the afternoon not returning to say goodbye to our guests.

This behaviour was totally out of character and was shocking to the family, as this outburst was in front of a group of friends. Later I realised that Fulton was now unable to cope in social gatherings. Fulton was not interested anymore in joining in these social occasions, and often walked outside, leaving our visitors inside to go to the security and safety of his outside domain. At this time, I thought he was being rude when he did this.

After the Dementia diagnosis, on reflection I realised that he had not been able to keep up the pace of conversation needed when engaging with our friends and family. Probably the plaque on his brain was already preventing him from understanding conversational chatter.

Fulton was still playing golf every Saturday. But much later I learned from Bill his golf partner that during a game, occasionally he would hit the ball then start to wander off in a fog of confusion, not knowing what he was supposed to do next. His friends were very loyal and did not confide in me. At that time, they were apparently aware of Fulton's changed behaviour. I think he also knew something was wrong, but again masked this problem as a way to cope with his own confusion.

Around that time, he had a minor operation on his leg and said he would take a break from golf. So he was able to mask his confusion about the game to his friends, by explaining he could not play for a while due to the operation.

He never played again but he continued to meet his friends for lunch after their golf game on a Saturday. Fulton was in the habit of joining me after golf for a coffee and chat with my friend Shirley at Manuka in the late afternoon, before going back home to the farm. These were happy times full of idle chatter and laughter or serious talks when we tried to solve the problems of the world.

Then one day Shirley said, 'Isn't that Fulton sitting at the cafe next door?'

I was nonplussed by this and said to Shirley, 'I guess he didn't see us. I'll let him know we are here,' so I wandered over to where he was sitting sipping a milkshake.

'Hi, how was golf? Didn't you see us? We're just over there.'

'I know,' he replied with annoyance, 'I'm tired I don't want to talk to you both now!'

Fortunately, Shirley who had been a friend for over thirty years did not take offence at Fulton's obvious desire to sit alone. Again, I accepted his personality change as part of the ageing process. Although I was embarrassed by this episode, it was only the beginning of a series of indications that Fulton had Dementia. But two years were to pass, and the peculiar behaviours increased, before we received a definitive medical diagnosis.

One such bizarre incident marked a crossroads for me. After this happened, I knew something was drastically wrong with Fulton, and I would have to convince him to see his doctor. That was an extremely difficult thing to do as he had always avoided seeking medical advice for himself. But after this experience even he admitted something was seriously wrong and needed to be addressed.

During a severe thunderstorm, I phoned him at work to tell him the flood waters were rising and our farm would be cut off from the main road within an hour. He told me I was exaggerating the situation, and he would come home when he wanted to do so. The police were issuing warnings over the radio and local TV station to let residents know the road would be closed shortly. I passed on these updates to him, but my ensuing pleas to Fulton again fell on deaf ears. He said he would come when he had finished his work and that as he had been commuting from our farm to his office for over twenty years, he was the best judge of the road, not some TV reporter!

Eventually, after a couple of hours had elapsed, I decided to check on the flooding at our front gate. Hopefully he was down at the gate waiting to get through the water as it usually dropped after a few hours. It was still raining heavily, but in the darkness I could see the flashing lights at our gates indicating the police were still at the roadblock they had set up to alert motorists to turn back to the main road.

When I asked them to let me know when Fulton arrived there, one police officer said, 'Oh, yes, we remember him. He was here an hour ago. He ignored all our directions and drove straight through the barriers and crashed into the water. Don't worry, we managed to pull him out of the car through the window. He is not injured, just very annoyed and wet! You can arrange to get the car towed out of the water tomorrow. Phone the SES. Your husband has been taken into the Queanbeyan evacuation community centre.'

I was shocked and embarrassed to hear this and I was shaking as I splashed back up our road, in the torrential rain, to tell the children their father had been involved in an accident but was safe. Why had he ignored the barricades, flashing lights and the police signalling him to stop?

When I finally spoke to Fulton on the phone later that night he made no sense at all. I tried desperately to understand him but he was speaking gobbledygook. Eventually a rescue worker took the phone and explained to me that Fulton was disoriented, partially dressed, and refusing offers of dry clothing! He was marooned in town, cut off from us, and we could not reach him until the flood waters receded.

It was a scary situation but he was brought home the following day by a kind SES worker, who told us Fulton might be suffering from shock!

When this drama was over Fulton could not explain or remember what had happened, but insisted he needed to go to work the following day.

But at last, after this incident, common sense prevailed – and I managed to convince him to see his doctor immediately.

This certainly had not been normal behaviour and Fulton at last recognised something was wrong. His GP was a friend of over forty years, he and his wife and family had become close family friends. I phoned him privately and relayed the story about the flood and the litany of symptoms Fulton had been exhibiting prior to his accident in the storm. We went together to see the doctor the following morning and at last he recommended Fulton see a specialist for some blood tests and hopefully a diagnosis.

Surprisingly, the specialist said Fulton had prostate cancer and that was possibly the cause of his personality change, because of the hormonal changes! I very much doubted that was all that was affecting Fulton and felt there was something else really wrong with his thinking and cognitive ability, which would possibly require more medical testing in the future. The good news was that Fulton finally decided he would retire soon and agreed to do some overseas travel. Over the next year he did receive ongoing treatment for the prostrate cancer but refused to have surgery.

I hoped for a miracle as I wanted Fulton to be able to relax and enjoy the next years as peacefully as possible. However, I did not see any improvement at all in his peculiar behavioural antics, but rather a deterioration in his cognitive ability and an escalation in his odd behaviours.

We decided to sell the farm as soon as possible so we could move closer to town as it was becoming increasingly difficult to manage the many trips to doctors and hospital from such a distance. Fulton argued with me throughout each trip into town saying that I was panicking and he did not need to see a doctor. I retired from my volunteer work so we could spend more time together and persuaded Fulton it was time to relax and smell the roses. At last he agreed.

We spent a couple of months organising the farm for sale. This was a period of sustained total disaster as far as Fulton was concerned. He ranted and raved about not wanting to leave the farm and continually undermined my efforts to pack up forty years of family living.

Although he had agreed to the sale, he became totally obstructionist, unpacking boxes I had packed, hiding precious jewellery and family treasures, 'in case they might be stolen by the removalists'.

I found a string of pearls, a twenty-fifth wedding anniversary gift, five years after he had passed away, cleverly hidden at the back of a bureau drawer which had been moved to our beach house after we sold the farm. This was long after I had given up hope of ever finding them.

Our family home was rather big, having numerous bedrooms, formal living rooms, large conservatory with a sunken spa, pool and tennis court. At the far end of our home there was a self-contained flat.

Packing up a home that large would be a big job for anyone, but in my situation it was extremely difficult. My 'helper' seemed to be on a series of daily missions which had no rhyme or reason. He might unpack boxes in the garages and spread the contents all over the gardens. He would hide himself in his study and spend hours fossicking in the filing cabinet, then distribute the files into the empty cupboards in the flat.

At weekends the children helped me in this mammoth job and all agreed, that 'Dad is trying to stop the move by his antics'. He moved dozens of planters from the garden and packed them carefully into the empty spa, and so it went on.

At the time I thought he was waiting for me to say, 'I give up – we will not sell the farm, we don't need to move.' But I knew I just had to keep going, trying to keep ahead of Fulton's delaying tactics.

After the Dementia diagnosis, I realised he just did not know how to help me pack up the house to sell the farm.

Not long after selling the farm, we had our last trip down to our beach house at Malua Bay. That had its bittersweet moments, but we all enjoyed just being together as a family walking on the beach in the late afternoon, as the sun was setting. Fulton was at his happiest sitting at our big dining room table playing Trivial Pursuit with us all gathered around, a game he had always enjoyed. We played in pairs.

Fulton however no longer understood the questions but constantly said, 'I know the answer to this one.' We all laughed together a lot during that last game, and he probably laughed the most. Fulton had always been competitive in whatever sport or game he was playing. He had always been very good at the history answers and questions in Trivial Pursuit. So that last time we used the history questions.

No matter what question was asked, like 'What was the name of Henry VIII's first wife?', he would confidently answer, 'I know the answer to that one. It's USSR! See, you can't trip me up.' That evening we played for a long time with Fulton excitedly calling out 'USSR' to all the questions. We all enjoyed that game as much, probably more than any other we had ever played.

So although his mind was rapidly deteriorating, we were still able to experience happy family gatherings. But sadly this was not for long.

After moving out of the farm and before we took up residence in our new home in Canberra, I booked a favourite apartment overlooking the beach on the Gold Coast. Some of the family lived up there permanently, and I arranged this holiday so all the children could enjoy a holiday together with their father. Although our children were all adults by this time, we enjoyed the idea of coming together for a family holiday.

At that time none of us knew it would be our last family holiday with Fulton. One night I invited Fulton's old school mate Macca and his wife Jan to join us all for dinner. I thought Fulton might be able to still do some of his bar-tending tasks. How wrong I was. The children were in charge of the barbeque. I had set up the glasses, the gin, tonic, beer and wine on the bench.

Macca asked Fulton for a G&T. By the bewildered look on Fulton's face, I realised then he had no idea what to do. I quickly handed him the gin and put the bottle of tonic within easy reach. Fulton took the gin and poured a full glass! Macca went over and said, 'Leave it to me Mouldy, I'll take over now.'

Later Macca said to me, 'Poor Mouldy, he's no good is he?'

It was the following morning that Fulton collapsed beside us on the grass as we walked home from a family breakfast at our favourite Broadbeach restaurant. He lay there for a few seconds, opened his eyes and looked at our worried faces in surprise. He then stood up with our help and said, 'These bloody shoes, I'm throwing them out when I get home.'

He again refused to see a doctor but rather blamed the 'stupid' new shoes I had bought for him. So despite all of our concerns, I decided nothing would be gained by arguing with Fulton there.

After a few heated discussions with all the children, Fulton finally agreed to see his doctor as soon as we returned to Canberra. We all knew now something was seriously wrong with Fulton this time, but decided to try to relax and enjoy the remainder of our family holiday up north. Fulton swam, walked on the beach, and sat with us on the balcony watching the sun go down, whilst sipping his favourite G&T. He hardly spoke but seemed happy just to sit and listen to the family chatting.

After consulting our family doctor as soon as we returned to Canberra, the actual diagnosis was really an anticlimax. We had known for a long time that something was seriously amiss with Fulton. Despite our attempts to determine what was causing these changes in his behaviour, the GP felt that prostrate cancer was the primary cause. However now it appeared obvious that something more insidious was the reason. We went together to our GP and again related his litany of symptoms, adding details of his recent collapse.

Thankfully this time our doctor referred Fulton to a gerontologist who requested he have an MRI. One week later we returned to her office and I was thinking that at last we might receive a diagnosis. We sat in her office and she said, 'Fulton, you have plaque on your brain which is consistent with you having Dementia with Lewy Bodies.'

She then turned to me and said in a matter of fact voice, 'Mrs Muir, you have a window of about three months, should you wish to travel before it becomes too difficult.' She added, 'It might be a good idea to hide all your sharp knives!'

Just as well we were both pragmatic people, as the delivery of Fulton's diagnosis certainly was not sugarcoated!

She may have said something else but I did not hear anything as I believe I was in shock. I had prepared myself for a stroke diagnosis or a brain tumour. But Dementia ... about which I knew very little. What next? What should we do? In the car driving home, Fulton commented rather drily, 'Now you know why I did not want to consult a doctor. They only deliver bad news!' He had lost so much cognition but not his sense of humour. I realised at this moment I became Fulton's carer and our true Dementia journey began.

After this definitive diagnosis of Dementia with Lewy Bodies, our children were dealing with their own grief at slowly losing their father to this disease. We both had tried in our own ways not to burden them any further with our grief and despair. It had been much easier talking to them about the prostate cancer diagnosis because we all knew what treatment and prognosis was involved.

A Dementia with Lewy Bodies diagnosis hit us all like a volcanic explosion.

I did not need to ask the family for their support and assistance. They were all supportive from the start. I really appreciated that they rallied around and helped us along the journey. In fact, I tried to encourage all the children to make the most of the time they had left with their father. We had family lunches and dinners, and our children all tried in their own way to spend quality time alone with their father.

Alycia, who was recently married and living in Sydney, put her doctoral studies on hold, and moved back from Sydney to stay with us so she could spend time with Fulton and assist me in caring for him. Her husband Olli remained in Sydney for work and commuted to Canberra at weekends. It was a tough time for Alycia but having her at home meant a great deal to

Fulton and myself. More importantly it gave Alycia precious time with her father.

I am sure it was very hard for her to see on a daily basis how her father was rapidly changing. However we did have some fun times sitting after the evening meal as she tried to decipher some of the historical records she was working on for her research. It surprised me that Fulton had the ability to decipher some of the copperplate writing. Yet in other regards he was showing rapid deterioration in his cognitive ability.

Initially Olli was commuting at weekends but eventually they moved to Canberra and Olli worked remotely, only going to Sydney once a fortnight. I am sure not all employers would be as supportive as Olli's were.

Fiona spent almost every weekend with her father, taking him for walks, to lunch or to a movie. Most of the time he was totally oblivious to the reason behind these outings but Fiona certainly enjoyed her special time with her father. That is not to say she was not challenged from time to time by his lack of social boundaries and difficult temperamental outbursts!

I arranged for Fulton to fly up north to have a couple of mini-breaks with his daughter Melinda, her husband John and her brother Jonathon, while he still was mentally able to cope with travelling, albeit with much support from the airline. He enjoyed these holidays, which provided me with brief respite from my caring role.

While he was away, I was free each day to visit and assess the suitability of the local nursing homes in Canberra, as I knew Fulton would need full-time care in the future. I was resisting this idea, but in my heart I knew it would become a reality I could no longer ignore.

I had encouraged Fulton to fly up to the Gold Coast to spend time with Melinda before Dementia took over completely. It also enabled Melinda and the family to experience living with Fulton when he was in the mid-stage of the disease. Melinda learned to help Fulton with his dressing after his first day there, when he tried to dress himself in John's clothes which were far too big for him. Spending quality time alone with her father was something I know she appreciated.

Fulton often appeared confused now and was totally bewildered by social occasions in which he previously had been totally at ease. Now he seemed to be like a ship without its rudder.

He was confused in group situations. Talking one-to-one was easier for him to cope with.

Bianca and her children often popped in for short visits after school which Fulton and I really enjoyed. We shared a cup of tea and a chat whilst the children took Edith for a walk around the block. Somehow the lively chatter and natural joy of the children cheered us both up immensely.

Some days they came for a longer visit when Fulton even managed to play hide and seek with Millie and Liam at the local park. We all would walk up to the park at the end of our block to play. We nominated the seat there as our 'whippy' and the many large trees provided excellent hiding spots for the children. On a couple of occasions Fulton only counted to three before turning around to start to walk home alone, forgetting that the children were still hiding up a tree, waiting to be discovered. The children would call out to Fulton that he had forgotten to find them. However he was off in his own world, oblivious of leaving the children wondering as to why he was leaving them and not finishing the game.

They agreed Fulton was a bit funny, but were not at all worried by his non-engagement, in fact his behaviour just made them laugh. Our other children were all wonderful helping me in many ways, sometimes just sitting with him at home, or coming in the car to help Fulton be safe and making sure he did not open the door whilst the car was in motion. Every small assistance I appreciated so much.

These memories, good, funny and sad, which the children experienced with him over this period, were to be the last they would have of their father. So the diagnosis did not prevent Fulton participating in family events, but now he often appeared lost and confused. He was present in body, but his mind was totally absent.

Glimpses of his great mind and sense of humour surprisingly made fleeting appearances. But sadly the man I married and the children's father had diminished into the shadows of the disease which engulfed him.

I tried to ensure he was never alone and certainly endeavoured to include him in as many family gatherings as possible. However other social events were curtailed as his cognitive ability diminished.

His diagnosis marked the beginning of a new part of our journey. Living together as carer and husband.

BLANCHE AND JACK'S STORY

Dear Jenny
I fully agree it was wasted time, but something good has come from our journey to help other carers.

I still live in frustration thinking of our merry-go-round of visits to a team of medical experts, searching for a clinical diagnosis that lasted for several years, with no definitive outcome ...

***

When Jenny and I first started talking about writing this book, we reflected for a long time and asked ourselves: What are the important Dementia stories we need to tell? What were the obstacles we struggled and what helped? How did we learn to accept the uncertainty of the illness? And why did we draw on the topics we are now addressing in our Dementia writings?

In our writings, we amplify our voices and highlight the stories that had a memorable and devastating impact on our caring roles. Now we wish that through our writings our message is seen as powerful, as we walk with our readers to share some of the stories that helped, informed and inspired us to understand Dementia.

Today Jenny's and my relationship has moved from the therapeutic peer support we both craved at the time, to a relationship that is evolving into a strong friendship!

We hope by reading our real lived Dementia stories as carers for our husbands, our Dementia experience will help you to gain a better Dementia knowledge to understand the illness through our experiences. And, like me, take the opportunity to access the community support readily available from experts in the field. The support I received has left an indelible mark, so much so that I want others to benefit similarly. May our independent stories also be another objective perspective as a resource tool?

Jack and I worked in tandem to consider what treatment options we had available, to halt the progressive memory loss that had started to affect our way of life. We found ourselves waiting for treatment options for years, filled with desperate hope. Together we spent countless hours in doctor's surgeries, hospital waiting rooms, specialist clinics repeatedly explaining Jack's health history and his medication regimen. In the process of this search, we spent many thousands of dollars.

It is hard to actually pinpoint with absolute certainty when I first noticed the early triggers that something was not quite right with Jack's memory lapses. Thinking, knowing, remembering, decision-making letdowns became noticeable, when Jack received an unforeseen redundancy notice along with other senior colleagues.

This unforeseen job loss unravelled not only his confidence, but it affected his personality as well. Slowly the dark clouds started to form, and he became mentally and physically restless. I readily accepted this new behaviour as apparent signs of explicit grief and pain. For my husband, who was a senior accountant and closely associated with the organisation for 25 years, the financial loss was not the focus, rather a life-changing decision had been taken on his behalf. And Jack had failed to see the signs.

Jack took immense pride in his independent nature which he conscientiously cultivated over the years: his 'I can do it, fix it, manage it, figure it' attitude. He willingly accepted challenges, often saying, 'I'm bigger than the job itself,' no matter how daunting the task and in good grace he would often figure solutions to solve them. Yet it was beyond him now to find a workable solution for his job loss.

Unlike Dementia symptoms, depression is easy to manage with prescription medication. Jack having accepted a new consultancy position with the same organisation, his mood lifted and he immersed himself in his job again.

The new consultancy position had more flexibility and made less demands on his time and he was determined to halt the depressive thoughts taking hold, by not seeing his permanent job loss as a tragedy but a change of lifestyle. Instead he started to design a more constructive time plan to study 'depression' through various mediums to empower himself. Reading other people's stories enabled him to glean from them an understanding that he was not alone suffering depression. That gave him immense comfort and relief that, despite depression, he could still easily engage in the endless opportunities on offer.

Now that he was again in control of his work schedule, he enthusiastically looked forward to work–life balance, and adopted positive measures and they became his 'magic pill' for another ten years of full-time employment.

The above experiences show depression leading to memory issues in the early stages of Dementia are subtle and a sufferer can still lead a full life. But, at the same time Jack craved people's attention to talk about his memory concerns and, even though in total conflict with his independent nature, it fitted perfectly with how Jack's mind worked before the Dementia diagnosis.

Jack would describe his depression symptoms like a 'fog in his brain' and if he tried to think 'his head hurt badly' and this is the perfect way to describe his 'fear'. This slow memory change, along with loss of control and stability, terrified Jack and he often felt helpless not knowing how to fix the problem.

Like Dementia, depression too can take on different forms and is unique how it plays out for each sufferer. So is the recovery. Also like Dementia, depression is hard to recognise in the early stages, until it is fully developed.

Loss of memory is more than forgetting a shopping list or the names of your family members. Jack in the early days showed subtle signs of anxiety and was unable to follow the practical routines around the home. We never possessed a stove-top kettle, but he had one growing up, and he started putting our electric kettle on the gas stove!

In the early days the Dementia symptoms were difficult to process, as the disease is not black-and-white and moves through many stages. There are no early intervention measures in place, like there are for people who have cancer.

Dementia works slowly but surely, and hits not only the memory, but affects emotions, the person begins to feel less useful, experiencing continual loss of basic skills. It takes years to manifest and for each person the Dementia experience plays out differently, all taking its toll on the person's character!

Dementia is a slow and progressive loss, that leaves many families unable to plan their remaining years. The daily loss of abilities takes years before it is obvious to carers. Especially as it takes the carer years to really understand and accept the rollercoaster of Dementia emotions – and still to date, there is little hope!

Jack's ability to rely on autopilot had become unreliable. He would forget to turn off the car's indicator when he moved lanes and had difficulties in reversing and parking. Even more scary, was when his reflexes became slow and he would fail to recognise familiar turn-offs, including important landmarks that had been part of his roadmap for years. Most annoying was his dismissive attitude to mask these events as a moment of distraction, saying, 'I can only do one thing at a time'.

Jack's physical and mental inabilities to function at a high level became visible to our family particularly when it required him to encompass language, imagination and perception. It was these endless memory failures which eroded his self-confidence and he was aware it was not a normal stage of the ageing process. He remarked, 'I am well aware that the human body starts to behave strangely with age, but in my case, my memory loss is failing me more often than is normal and it is time I got help.'

We all depend on our memory to get us from point A to B, and it is our memory that allows us to know who, what, where, when, why and how. But the Dementia process shrinks the brain and information relayed to the brain becomes disjointed, leading to detrimental effects on the important functions that we depend on, specifically emotions, speech, decision-making and sometimes even self-control.

Jack in the past would resolve any of his health problems by means of a good dialogue and looked for help tirelessly by self advocation and consultation with his GP. He started off with checking on his primary care health concerns and sometimes he was referred to specialists when his GP thought it was necessary.

In the early days before the Dementia diagnosis, Jack was still totally capable of self-advocacy and able to use his long-term memory of social skills to be 'on show' and perform successfully for a short duration of 10 to 20 minutes, as he always carried his trusty notes and referred to them endlessly. But if he was given a longer consultation, a very different scenario would unfold. At each of his medical visits he prepared specific questions to get answers to his memory fears and difficulties, although none were provided.

Jack disapproved altogether if I intervened with reassuring remarks, as he was desperate to remain in control and he made sure when in public not to reveal the 'nitty gritty' details of his memory loss difficulties, even with family, as he was mindful of not creating a negative image.

Writing about Jack's efforts to get an early diagnosis makes me feel guilty. I often sat and watched while he documented his medical history several times, only to be told by the medical staff that there was no real reason for his concern. We left each medical visit none the wiser, yet I found it strange we were instructed to return for another assessment in a few months' time.

After each of these medical visits Jack's moods would spiral to new lows, and I observed them in silence. Jack's aim was to understand and stop the self-doubts that were eroding his confidence, and not to attack or question the medical profession. My role was to watch from the sidelines and be his chauffeur. I was only encouraged to step in if a more accurate assessment was required. Slowly it became clear that I was not only a sole carer, but also a sole witness to the severe lack of early medical intervention measures for any sort for an early diagnosis. The continual memory loss only chipped at his confidence bit by bit, yet he suffered alone in solitary confinement of his own choosing.

My aim here is to highlight the lack of honest discussion we experienced with a range of medical practitioners.

We consulted to receive an early diagnosis, and I still fail to understand why we were not informed that memory loss can take years to diagnose and so why not have this conversation. Now I am aware that in order to find the cause, a patient has to go through several tests, to rule out specific causes, before a Dementia diagnosis can be delivered. The early treatments sometimes prescribed research has shown to have little benefit.

In spite of not receiving any relief for Jack's memory difficulties, his condition stayed relatively stable over a ten-year timeframe and he diligently managed to stay employed productively and still looked forward to our annual visits to see our daughter in London and his family in Holland.

In the early days, Jack kept a very detailed diary of his memory loss difficulties. They seriously undermined what he valued most: his independence, his dignity and his quality of life and he hoped the prepared questions would provide possible solutions:

- Why is my memory failing?
- What are the causes for my symptoms?
- Are there tests I can take?
- Is my memory loss temporary?
- Is it possible to stop further deterioration?
- Can memory loss and other health issues be managed together?

Carers and their families are sometimes faced with carrying a heavy burden of stigma and sometimes face barriers erected in the community to disempower carers. Old age beliefs in the healthcare industry exist that sometimes see a person with Dementia as unable to follow directions. This can result in poor physical therapy outcomes.

There is severe lack of Dementia education for the general public, and even are severely lacking for otherwise well-trained hospital staff. This can lead to a Dementia person being invisible, or visible only when a delusional episode is played out in public.

This is an event that our family experienced from a Dementia health professional, who despite her extensive training, was insensitive when Jack was slow to follow and understand what was required. But after the tests were completed, she remarked, 'Fancy – you have not lost your ability to use big words.'

This thoughtless remark was doubly sad, as I did not expect such a biased statement from a highly trained Dementia specialist. I see their role to improve the lives of people who are living with Dementia, and provide thoughtful and positive support for carers and their families. I do not know how Jack felt and thought it better not to discuss this incident. This little episode illustrates there is a pressing need for sensitivity training for Dementia staff.

In the past I never had a reason to keep an eye on Jack as he was a dependable and reliable operator and equipped to handle any challenges that came his way. But Dementia robbed Jack of his confidence and left him hesitant and indecisive. This behaviour in the early days often brought undue stress in our relationship.

I recall an incident, when I had to undergo a medical procedure at a day surgery. When he heard the news, Jack had a panic attack and our conversation reached a very irrational point that gave way to emotions with conflict arising.
I resolved this unreasonable dispute by agreeing to have our daughter Maria, who lived and worked in Darwin at the time,

come to Sydney for a 36-hour visit, to transport us to the hospital.

The imposition and the inconvenience on Maria's time did not concern Jack. It would have been a far cheaper option to take a taxi rather than pay for a return air ticket to Darwin. However I saw this behaviour again as Jack masking his inability to drive to the city and we both knew he was in no position to act in an emergency situation. To maintain peace, I found that I often agreed, as reasoned argument was now impossible.

The signs that he was unable to interpret signals were now extremely obvious. Like when the kettle boiled or when the washing machine had run its cycle. These everyday reminders made him extraordinarily obsessive and he talked frequently of his ongoing cognitive difficulties. He remarked, 'I recognise daily my once brilliant mind is now foggy, and it fails me more often than I like.'

Jack's on-going focus and conversation on his memory was like hearing a record stuck on a player and there was no dial that I could pick to move forward. Hearing such desperation pained me as it was beyond anyone to fix a diseased brain.

At both of our daughters' weddings, in 2004 and 2005, he began his father-of-the-bride speeches by waving his notes in the air saying, 'Sadly I need these notes as my memory is not what it used to be.' Jack's memory difficulties in the early days were not too obvious to others, yet very obvious to me and the family. Mr Perfectionist was unable to remember the name of the concert or opera he just attended, whereas in the past he would rattle off the name of the first violinist.

Methodical gardening skills now became erratic, although he still found great satisfaction and enjoyed the outdoors.

Despite the hours he spent in the garden, he now cultivated a robust weed patch, where once our kitchen produce flourished. Nonetheless generally being out of the house pottering and getting his hands dirty raised his spirits. It did not matter he watered the garden with a tangled hose. He got a huge kick pulling weeds with sadistic satisfaction, repotted plants and constantly moved pots from the front to the back garden. Our past predictable life was now more often 'unpredictable' and uncertainty now normal.

If I reminded him of our social commitments he would deny knowledge of them and instead accuse me of not giving him enough advanced notice. For instance, if I left a note for him to shop when I was at work, he would forget and cover his forgetfulness by masking his mistakes very skilfully.

Whilst I was on a solo visit to visit our daughter Jeannette in London, Jack burnt his food and threw kerosene on the pan, that started a small fire in the kitchen and he painted the whole kitchen to mask the accident – and did a good job in the bargain! Although on my return, he left traces of black ash in the corners of the kitchen cupboard. Jack's deceitful behaviours were new and I often wondered where to look for my wonderful husband who had disappeared, and I craved my old life!

Experiences like these are common and extremely difficult for carers as a Dementia sufferer can and does mask mistakes very well for a long time.

A methodical and detailed operator of the past had now disappeared and was replaced with a person who had more hits and misses than even a movie star cared to boast! Jack had reached a point where his past perfection was lost. He would still prepare the vegetables for our evening meal, but now he was unable to dice the vegetables evenly. I interpreted these behaviours to a teenager who is keen to run out to play. The frequency of his errors, I later learnt, were not designed to annoy me but the result of his faulty brain.

In 2005 when we both flew to London to attend Jeannette's wedding, the long plane trip was not a problem as Jack had slept for much of the way. But the landing was not as smooth. It took Jack a few days to adjust to the changed time zone, and we experienced several incidents. First, he left his wallet at security, then collected a wrong suitcase on the baggage reclaim and we had to turn around not only to return the wrong suitcase he collected but we had to find his. Finally on our way out on the escalator to the parking lot, he accidentally released his grip, and his suitcase rolled to the bottom, luckily there was no one injured. I then became more alert for obvious signs of tiredness knowing his brain was unable to adjust as easily to the different time zone!

Jack now seemed dismissive of most of his everyday living commitments. He even lost interest in playing with our two delightful toddler grandchildren, who we minded in our home twice a week. His memory would fail him, even though I had instructed him to keep an eye on the grandkids whilst I prepared lunch. Jack would at all times accompany the family to the park, but would not participate, but instead sit on the park bench and stare into the distance, unaware that he was there to play with his grandchildren.

When the Dementia diagnosis happened, I suddenly found myself as a carer with little understanding and untuned to the memory struggle that Jack faced daily and how the daily strain of living had affected all aspects of his life. I noticed he started to rely on his written notes frequently to jog his memory.

But this was an old habit, he always carried a notebook to document ideas as they came. When he drove to park at a shopping centre he would write detailed notes of the location, the entrance gate, numbering system, the colour code, or any signs he thought would assist him to get back to the car easily.

Later Jack lost his ability to understand how to use numbers, extremely sad as he had spent half his life working with figures. He would seek my help to prepare the exact liquid formula to feed plants or to prepare the pesticide sprays.

He also lost his ability to remember passwords, placing a list of login and password details under his desk mat and later unable to figure out the appropriate matches when required.

When you begin to understand the impacts of Dementia, you begin to realise why a person with Dementia is often frustrated, depressed and annoyed. A Dementia-impacted brain is unable to process information quickly, even though the brain is still functioning – and as a carer it takes a long time to accept and get accustomed to the daily loss that you witness each day.

Dementia is not only a memory problem, it is a devastating and terminal illness that unfortunately only gets worse. It affects emotions, personality and movement. The brain is a well-crafted complex machine and once broken, it is difficult to repair or put back together.

Even close to the Dementia diagnosis, Jack was totally able to use public transport to get to the city and find his way around and get home safely. Having stopped driving was no excuse to stay home.

I recall a conversation Maria had with her father, by simply asking 'Dad, would you be able to live with your conscience if you killed a young mother like me, especially as your driving reaction is as slow as your speed?' He took a literal note of this conversation and immediately stopped driving and never looked back, as long as his keys were left in the top drawer. Jack never showed any interest in cars – to him they were a mode of transport that took him from A to B.

For a long time even after the Dementia diagnosis, Jack continued to carry on with his daily walks unaccompanied, and only once was confronted with a roadblock that had him unsettled momentarily. He decided to continue, even though he lost his bearings and took a wrong turn. Yet he managed to get home safely without asking for help with directions. Exhausted but otherwise untroubled by the event.

Love is key. I cannot imagine what caring for a partner or family member with Dementia would be like if you had not had a loving relationship to begin with. Even though the person who you share your daily life is not the person you once knew, you simply keep going for the incredible memories accumulated over the decades together. He was a constant reminder why I had accepted and continued with the care role.

The early days are the hardest, and many marriages fail, as the person you live with becomes a stranger. I often felt like I wanted to get out of the marriage, to pack my bags and leave. Yet the time spent caring slowly taught me to learn to understand Dementia and to accept the relationship is no longer equal or shared. Pain, struggle and heartbreak are part of the journey and become a carer's burden.

Jack could no longer cope with social events and withdrew. He controlled his isolating behaviour with a closely guarded routine.

Dementia too is a body-mind-spirit disease, but unlike cancer and heart diseases, does not receive any physical support as there is no treatment for it. So it is left to the carer to manage the emotional and spiritual sides that arise. I often just muddled through when I first started the role of a carer.

Jack often became overwhelmed when his sensory stimulants became too much to cope at our special family celebrations. He was well aware his family yearned to have him socially engaged with his presence and this obligation to his family actually made him physically sick. So debilitating was his discomfort that he would bend down in pain holding on to his stomach. Over time it was obvious to the family he was unable to enjoy or participate in social events!

With the passing of time, Jack's Dementia progressed to new heights and I was unable to make sense of his scattered and confused thoughts, because Dementia was now slowly taking a hit on his brain and the brain was letting him down. His language difficulties severely contributed to his decision-making process and is clear proof that memory and language are bundled together.

In the later years of Jack's professional life, he dreaded office meetings, unable to understand the full gist of the conversation as voices came at him from all sides. At this point he was still fully aware that he was unable to express himself succinctly, once his pride. He resolved the difficulty of his meeting problems by resorting to face-to-face meetings, as he had started to lip read.

The use of a mobile phone was relatively new technology in the early days of his memory difficulties, and he was unable to learn a new skill, despite the effort he made. In the end he just gave up in frustration saying, 'Why bother? I have managed without mobiles for most of my working career, and see no reason to start now.' Again, Jack was masking his inability to learn new tasks.

His technical wizardry was also lost. Before he took care of all our media systems, now he was unable to operate a CD and video.

It was striking and sad, as Jack saw much of himself located in language, being fluent in four languages. An excellent communicator, even though English was not his first language. He could easily switch from one language to the next, and he enjoyed a good debate and was well skilled to express himself with words. Sensing this acute loss to interact with people pained him, and that rational debate to accurately forecast the future was lost. Jack became paranoid that his good name would be tarnished if his colleagues discovered his cognitive decline and, rather than have this happen, he decided to bow out gracefully.

It became obvious to Jack that it was time to take off the mask and relieve himself of the high stress that was part of his job and, with huge relief, he handed in his retirement notice and called it a day, when he turned 65!

Jack had communication difficulties with Jeannette who lived in London, as he was unable to sustain telephone or face-time to stay in touch. It was a pressure and stress he could not handle, and sadly, the gradual end of a loving and regular contact between father and daughter ended abruptly! Where once there was a close and lively contact.

Jeannette had to endure the pain of her father's illness from a great distance, and she knew she could not change the situation. Nevertheless Jeannette readily accepted her father's communication difficulties and it pained her that she was not part of the family inner circle to contribute to her father's comfort, or lessen the responsibilities for her mother and sister. So she resolved the tyranny of distance by coming home to Sydney every six months and kept the physical contact with her father. Jack even waited for her arrival from London before he took his last breath.

Besides, both our children were also mothers with young babies, who both juggled professional careers.

I also noticed when our children are together there is a pre-existing tension due to tiredness that surfaces easily. They had to adapt slowly to the loss of a loving father who, although alive, was gone. Gone too was their familiar lifestyle that had now shifted 'off-centre' adding to their frustration. Dementia had also robbed Jack of his ability to display emotions, and he regretted that he could not physically attend his sister's funeral in Holland in 2006, even though as children they shared a close bond.

Maria who lived in Sydney was more privy to the actual reality being medically trained. Yet it is no easy fate when faced as a daughter bearing the responsibility for her father's care alone, without the support of her sister. She had to be strong to accept her father's condition. Being able to connect with her father at some level displayed genuine love, and the love she had allowed her to cope with her own anxiety.

Despite our proactive measures, the family had no choice but we were forced to live and act with our emotions of fear, worry, horror, sorrow, anger, pity and terror. In the end it became our family's pain to watch Jack succumb to the devastating Dementia symptoms that slowly affected not only his memory but his physical strength.

A brilliant man struck down by a disease, he wrestled with many of life's challenges. The most undermining was his lost decision-making ability to retain independence that he most valued, along with his unique ability to be independent and solve complex problems as they surfaced.

This demonstrated the painful truth about the Dementia disease; that anyone is susceptible, no matter how brilliant, how important, or how virtuous. The brain plays a huge part in important daily functions, including voluntary movement and sensory perception. Jack had many falls as his Dementia progressed, his balance became shaky and weak, when he was up on his feet.

On our third and final visit with the neurologist, Jack was prescribed medication, and after only three weeks I noticed slight memory progress and as a result Jack displayed less confused moments and even less anxiety, and I wondered why this prescription medication had not been administered much earlier?

However I have subsequently learnt that Dementia is one of the most significant illnesses that the developed world faces today. Currently there is no effective treatment to prevent, to slow, or to manage the early symptoms due to the unpredictable situation of the Dementia disease and also insufficient government and private funding internationally.

To further complicate the Dementia problem, many sufferers have multiple conditions, including Jack who was diagnosed with Dementia, Lewy Body and to date there is no treatment that can target each of the specific symptoms that some Dementia patients endure. Jack's behaviour for part of the day was normal, he looked well, his walk would be normal, and then at other times he appeared totally confused, muddled or sleepy.

Jack's waking hours unsettled him due to the rush of the morning routine to leave the house on time to keep our several early medical or social appointments. Nor did Jack's inability to be remain optimistic help with the ongoing challenges around him. For instance, he detested that I invaded his space each morning, and he would have preferred to be left alone, and this dependency only amplified his loss. He blankly refused paid carers' help, as he saw them as strangers.

In spite of my constant presence, he knew full well there was little he could do, yet he never accepted the one thing most of us cherish: he could no longer self-determine his life. The ongoing dialogue whilst dressing, 'Stand up, sit down, first put on underpants and then trousers' became sounds he wanted turned off.

Later, I learnt from a matron-friend it is best to put the two items of clothing together and this way the person only has to lift himself once.

Looking back, Jack's Dementia journey was evident first with severe depression symptoms. Dementia affected all aspects of daily life. Food, sleep, debilitating fatigue, lack of concentration and occasional vivid hallucination occurred. Just as depression takes non-identical forms and is also difficult to recognise early, the process of change can take years to be apparent and noticeable signs only appear towards the end.

During this period we lived in the Lower Blue Mountains and Maria had just completed her Higher School Certificate, and Jeannette had already left home and lived in the city to be nearer to her work, university and the social hub. Now, with both children at Sydney universities, we too decided to leave the Blue Mountains and relocate to Sydney so that we could keep the children home a bit longer. This meant moving house. Jack showed little interest in our search for a new house and seemed happy that I took on the job and Jeannette offered to help. Yet our discussion would appear normal and reasonable if a house came on the market that ticked all the right boxes.

There is no denying a home move brings with it undue stress at the best of times, but for Jack the burden of a house move and to allocate the time to pack decades of our possessions was beyond his capabilities. I can see this now, but was unaware at the time I had assigned packing responsibilities for us both. However when the removalists arrived on that day, none of the boxes that Jack was assigned were packed, that we literally had to throw the garden furniture, plants and tools unboxed and unlabelled into the truck.

This was when I was finally hit by the reality that the man I had known for over 25 years was becoming unreliable and unpredictable, and that was not the Jack I knew. Jack and I always worked well and were good judge of each other's work ethics. In all our time together, I cannot recall a time when I ever had to check or remind Jack of his responsibility.

Whereas now in hindsight with better Dementia understanding, Jack's lack of attention to detail was the result of his early signs of Dementia taking a slow grip and, over the years, frequent disruptive changes occurred on a regular basis. Where once there was calm, now there was chaos, instead of peace there was daily exhaustion, and instead of timelines I had to rush!

In this slow and long Dementia path, the damage to the brain is already taking place at a continuous steady slow pace. It is difficult to recognise the first sign of memory loss as the symptoms are not clearly defined or simply not consistent to set the alarm, there are signs of danger ahead, especially as I simply put them down as senior moments!

Dementia is common in our society. Memory loss affects all aspect of a patient's daily life and their families. Making it hard for families affected to receive the diagnosis positively, as there is still stigma attached. How I wish now that I had spent more time trying to understand Dementia rather than spending countless hours trying to find a cure.

Dementia education only began when Jack was delivered the Dementia diagnosis. Before this I was largely ignorant and muddled along in frustration. That added further stress because of the precarious uncertainty of our lives. I had no idea that science had not found a cure and when the disease was confirmed.

A person with early and middle stages of Dementia does not look sick, like people with cancer, until the very end of the Dementia illness. I often found myself reflecting in the early days as his carer, if Jack was really unaware of the effect his behaviour had on our relationship, because one minute he displayed total confidence and within minutes I was dealing with a changed character who was confused and muddled.

I recall in the early days I was never relaxed when Jack was behind the wheel, even though he would ask me to relax. Now that I have had a little exposure to Dementia education, I am well aware that no amount of coaching or yelling would have helped in the early days. I now regret why I allowed myself to get so exhausted daily. I now wish I had learnt to dance in the rain rather than worry about the storm ahead. For a long time, the family and friends did not recognise that anything was wrong, even when Jack demonstrated strange moments.

After years of visiting several clinics to get a cure, we soon learnt there is no one single test that can correctly give a Dementia diagnosis, so for years we went through a number of tests to actually pinpoint Jack's memory problems. Tests carried out were as follows: full cognition, blood and laboratory, MRI, CT and neuropsychological assessments.

In Jack's case it took a clinical psychologist, a clinical neuropsychologist and three visits to the neurologist to make the final Dementia Lewy Body diagnosis.

Jack had always been extremely proactive with his regular visits to his GP who managed his primary health, including his existing chronic diseases.

The Mini-Mental State Exam (MMSE) test gave a rough estimate of Jack's cognitive losses, his ongoing problem with inattentiveness, language difficulties and emotional changes. I accompanied Jack when he did these tests to provide additional information when Jack was unable to recall.

Yearly blood tests were taken to detect any other physical problems like an active thyroid gland and diabetes. Both these tests came back negative. However the Vitamin B-12 deficiency test came back positive and Jack was treated with B-12 injections twice a year.

As Jack's dementia advanced, he was prone to regular bouts of urinary tract infections (UTIs) that is common for some Dementia suffers, and it is important that antibiotic treatment is prescribed with some urgency. If not, severe infection sets in, exhibiting sudden confusion and delirium, along with withdrawal symptoms.

A routine blood test to check the health of Jack's prostate came back positive and he underwent surgery in 2008 and he experienced a delusional attack whilst he was still on the operating table shouting the Nazis were out to get him and he could see people on the wall aiming their guns at him.

The surgeon after a few days whilst he was recuperating at the hospital organised for Jack to be screened for a magnetic resonance imaging (MRI), to detect if anything else was occurring in his brain. Radiological findings often detect specific neurodegenerative disorders and these radiological findings are necessary to confirm the diagnosis. But the MRI results came out clear and the surgeon put the episode as an anaesthetic reaction, yet the hallucinations still continued for another few days whilst Jack was still in the hospital ward.

After Jack recovered from his surgery his GP requested more scans to rule out any further evidence of a stroke, bleeding, brain tumours or increased pressure due to fluids in the brain.

MRI testing, although non-invasive, can be extremely stressful for the staff when they have to deal with Dementia patients and their families. When Jack was taken into the confined, unfamiliar darkened room and settled in the unit, he panicked when he saw he was left alone, and started to move. Jack became unsettled and demonstrated anxiety, restlessness and refused to cooperate. The hospital medical staff were insufficiently trained in Dementia understanding to handle such patients. The goal of the MRI staff is to efficiently and effectively screen their patients but a Dementia patient does not understand the process, and they often delay the smooth operation of the unit.

I had accompanied Jack to the hospital's radiology unit in 2008, when the surgeon decided that he should have his first MRI to rule out other causes and Jack had no issue with the procedure. However in 2010 Jack was living at a nursing home and he had to have another MRI to ascertain his numerous falls. But when I picked Jack up from the nursing home he thought I was taking him home and he refused to cooperate to enter the hospital, and felt severely cheated. I had expected a challenge and had requested Maria's help to step in as I knew I could not manage him on my own. Maria noticed Jack's distress, and she approached the MRI staff and enquired, 'How can we all work together, to get the MRIs completed efficiently so we can all go home without any added stress?'

Here is a lesson – that a right approach can and does work!

Jack had two MRIs, yet over the two years, there was no noticeable signs of any abnormalities or functional changes. This is another indication that the Dementia disease is a mix of multiple symptoms, manifesting simultaneously in the brain, and the brain is actually fighting a long battle, being attacked for several decades before anyone is aware of the total break down.

After several years living with Dementia caring experience, I discovered that medical treatments vary from person to person and are specifically tailored and sometimes the treatment is combined to meet the required needs of an individual. The brain is a unique, intricate, elaborate and very delicate instrument, and to figure out the trial treatments that work or do not, is a long drawn-out process.

The most stressful aspect for a care giver were the years spent, living with the uncertainty of the disease. At each of our medical visits, I expected a definitive Dementia diagnosis which did not happen with no explanation given, yet we still had to continue, to invest our time, energy and finances, for outcomes that were vague.

I cannot stress enough the positive outcomes I acquired when I attended the carers' support groups in the local community for 2.5 hours that ran weekly. From the start, the commonality of our circumstances was felt, and it was a comfort to share, question, critique equally and loudly. The structure of this group was both informal and also the discussion was specifically targeted each week with expert talks to guide us carers, to foster a friendly carer's community and to solve mutual issues of concern that had become the carer's daily struggles.

These meetings were designed to assist carers to understand Dementia and to accept the disease for what it is and to accept the care role for what it was. It was only possible to attend this group meeting because Jack agreed to attend a daycare centre for five days a week.

Joining the group gave me the opportunity to feel validated, heard and understood. We were given access to other carers stories who were in a similar situation. There was laughter with funny Dementia stories being told – and the choice was always up to the carers to decide how much of their experiences they wished to share. The coordinator strongly encouraged carers to discuss their loneliness and the isolation they felt, and being carers without any training.

There was also the added bonus to hear professional Dementia speakers explain the Dementia process in simple language that empowered carers to learn and understand the disease in a safe and secure environment. It was also at these group meetings that I learnt of the ready resources available in the community, designed to lighten a carer's load each day.

It was the audiologist who subtly directed us to see the neurologist again, as Jack's follow-up hearing test results concerned the audiologist. These audio tests are generally non-invasive and painless and were carried out in a well-padded booth where the audiologist communicates with the patients via headphones, with clear instructions to follow varying tones, pitches played at different volumes and Jack was instructed to press a button when he heard or followed a sound or instruction.

However for Jack who had both hearing and cognition problems, his hearing test results were extremely unsatisfactory and at first suggested that I should consider an update. I immediately rejected this offer, and stated I was unwilling to invest in more top-of-the-range hearing aids as the ones we bought three years previously did not deliver the results we had expected. I also talked to her about my conversational experience with my neighbours, for whom English was their second language, and despite this, my conversation with both of them was far superior and engaging than it was with Jack. This experience demonstrated that it is simply impossible to separate audition and cognition and I was informed that impaired hearing difficulties can sometimes be a result of a neurological disorder.

However, as Jack's hearing or possibly his language understanding became more difficult, social interaction became a bigger barrier. He literally avoided most social contact with people that I initiated. When friends came to visit, he would interact for a short period, and would quietly disappear when he saw an opportunity. He also avoided staying home when I had book club meetings.

Jack was only comfortable in his familiar surroundings. He now preferred Maria to visit us in our home. It was a difficult task to find ways to maintain or strengthen his social connection with his daughters, his family and friends. When we had visitors, he occupied himself in the kitchen or the garden. One time when his brother Alphons was visiting from Holland, he politely pointed out to Jack that he should socialise with his guests rather than sit by himself in the kitchen, and Jack responded, 'I am unable to start the conversation.' His brother advised him 'to sit there and someone will come and talk'!

Even my efforts to encourage him to accompany me to the movies or concerts were mostly refused. Before his hearing loss, he thoroughly enjoyed going. Whereas before music did something special to his brain, he got his when he heard his favourite collections of music.

On the advice of the audiologist, I made our second appointment to see the neurologist, While the neurologist physically examined Jack, I took on another role. I found myself become a translator of sorts for Jack, as I was his support and helped him to connect and share his experiences. During this visit I was asked more specific targeted questions about Jack's current symptoms in order to figure how far his impairment had shifted from our last visit. And about his cognitive functions, behaviour and decision-making processes and if they had started to affect other aspects of his daily living.

Surely, I thought, this time I would get a definite diagnosis of some sort.

For instance, if Jack had cancer, all the tests he had already performed would have guided the doctor towards one illness or another. But for a dementia sufferer, the numerous tests that Jack underwent before the actual diagnosis, gave us no definitive results. We felt we were riding a medical merry-go-round and it was a very frustrating experience!

Jack was having significant trouble following all forms of communication, be it auditory or written, and would just go through the motions. As an example, he just went through the motion of turning the pages of the newspaper each morning at the breakfast table. In the old days he would have started his reading by lifting out the business supplement.

I sought clinical psychological help privately, as I was concerned with his profound memory loss. He was now unable to dress independently, unable to engage with family and friends socially, and so together we agreed to undergo a thorough cognitive evaluation. Tests of mental function are considered very important in a Dementia diagnosis process. The assessment findings were consistent with early stages of a neurodegenerative disorder. Again, no precise diagnosis was made, but the report findings gave us an objective baseline to evaluate his cognitive strength and weakness.

With the clinical psychologist's report, I made our third appointment to see the neurologist in 2011. The neurologist assessed the clinical psychologist's findings, which looked at Jack's past history, his current presentation and his cognitive tests.

The neurologist then informed us that neuropsychiatric symptoms are not uncommon at any stage of memory loss, and it was necessary to complete one more assessment test. Jack was referred for one more clinical neuropsychologist's test.

Again, Jack's memory, language, visual perception, attention, problem-solving, movement, senses, balance, reflexes were all evaluated. The clinical neuropsychologists again tested to rule out any other varieties of common medical events that sometimes can mimic cognitive issues and can look like Dementia, but that do respond to prescription medications. The most common of these is depression, or pseudo-dementia.

Jack again had to perform extensive assessment tests. These tests would also take into account the earlier findings of the clinical psychologist's report to track other cognitive disorders.

Weeks later, when we came to receive the assessment test results, we were contained in the doctor's room, with no sound of the outside world entering, and we sat silently waiting to hear the test results. I could think of no questions that would clarify my new fear, and my anger faded away.

The neurologist read the clinical neuropsychologist's test findings. In the light of Jack's past and present history of cognitive decline, his fluctuating alertness, confusion, word-finding difficulty and inability to follow conversation, the neurologist concluded that Jack certainly had cognitive impairment, which was enough to affect his memory function and Jack could be classified as having Dementia.

We were both very shattered with the Dementia diagnosis. In spite of not expecting a positive result, nothing would have actually prepared us to receive a positive result.

I sat captive in a vacuum of thought, numb with unbearable sadness on hearing the Dementia diagnosis. The doctor's voice faded further in the emptiness. Fragments of our lives exploded in my mind now, vividly projecting years of Jack's memory difficulties.

One particular incident surfaced. We had just picked up a new car, when heavy rain made driving difficult with poor vision of the road ahead. Jack had pulled to the side of the road to read the instruction manual and was unable to follow the instructions for how to turn on the windscreen wipers. Just as the rain puddles gathered around us, the cognitive difficulties I faced also pooled around.

A Dementia diagnosis is tough. It is made efficiently and effectively with little time spent to explain the diagnosis, given the limited consultation time we had with the neurologist. Support, resources and time are delivered at a later date by your GP and various community support groups.

The Dementia path is long and slow, but this was only the first base. There's a long road ahead as neither our life nor the Dementia path ends here. This was just another chapter.
The neurologist then dictated a letter to Jack's GP to inform him of the Dementia diagnosis and requested the GP provide us with early education and support, and direct us to Dementia resources in our local area.

For Jack the Dementia diagnosis came after years of torment, fear and dread with his increasing memory loss.
It is very sad.

Most people cannot even tell you what the word 'dementia' means. The illness is characterised by a decline in cognitive function, memory loss, confusion, disorientation, with difficulty communicating, reasoning, and planning. These are all symptoms of Dementia and Jack's last test results had just confirmed these symptoms.

It strikes you that there is still no escape from the sadness and loneliness. You regret that time has gone by with things unsaid, as in the last few years the equality in our relationship changed drastically and the companionship had become just one-sided!

It was difficult to acknowledge the end is near. Life with Dementia is a life on the run. There is little time for reflection that we were now living the autumn of our life and our time together had a very definite end date.

Jack's Dementia diagnosis tests began in 2008 and the Dementia diagnosis was only confirmed in 2011. With burning eyes, I controlled my tears from flowing freely and felt something inside my chest compress tighter and tighter, as Jack and I stood up to leave the doctor's rooms. We shook hands and left silently. We were again instructed to come back after several months for another checkup.

Now that we were safely buckled in our car, we drove home in companionable silence. I turned on the ignition and veered the car towards the hospital exit, numbed to fate until I reached home and, with a heavy grief-stricken heart, called our daughters with the sad news.

The search for an early diagnosis of some sort for Jack's memory loss had a huge impact on both our well-being for years. It was also a huge financial outlay. In spite of having private health insurance, with the cost of medical visits – especially specialist visits and screenings – the refunds from both Medicare and private health cover do not meet the costs invested.

Another important point is that the carer goes into Dementia care with little or no knowledge of Dementia symptoms, until after a diagnosis is delivered. The tailored Dementia courses, although very useful, are denied you until a carer has proof that a Dementia diagnosis has been delivered. In the meantime, carers have to live and muddle through with the illness for years without help.

***

Jenny and Blanche's tips:
Diagnosis journey

- Seek medical advice as soon as changes in behaviour occur.
- Ask for a second opinion if you are concerned about any aspect of a diagnosis.
- Ensure your financial situation is in order.
- Arrange to meet with your lawyer to ensure that all legal matters – including Power of Attorney and Will – are settled prior to any definitive diagnosis by a doctor is made, so that they are valid.
- Call a family meeting with a clear and realistic agenda and specifically ask for help. If a member of the family lives overseas, ask them to contribute financially to paid help around the home.
- It helps to take a deep breath when a situation becomes difficult. Walk out to the garden. Fresh air and scenery is magical – making you refreshed again with new energy to cope with the situation.
- You can count on being supported by genuinely caring community services and activities will be centred around individual needs, interests and choices.

Chapter 2

Caring at home

Understand, learn and accept

JENNY AND FULTON'S STORY

Dear Blanche
Walking on eggshells trying to navigate the mood swings and irrational outbursts was the story of my life for two years. Navigating a day as Fulton's carer required a rigid schedule mixed with structured activities and a large dose of patience and compassion ...

***

Usually, the care of a person with Dementia depends on the willingness of their partner or family to take on the role of primary carer. In the early stages, after the initial diagnosis, the primary carer needs the most support and information on what may lie ahead. They need to learn how to undertake the caring role.

As Fulton's carer, I had little success in learning exactly what this role would encompass.

Dementia develops in so many ways according to the type of Dementia which has been diagnosed. I think there are about 14 types of Dementia, all having different characteristics.

Blanche and I have written about how we cared for our husbands who were diagnosed with Dementia with Lewy Bodies. Despite this shared diagnosis, it is important to keep in mind that our journeys were unique, as were our husbands' needs.

Dementia caring is hard work and I believe there is no preparation or training that can completely alleviate the burden a carer carries on a daily basis. It may be particularly challenging to care for your partner or close family member, as you may have no choice in taking on this role because nobody else is available. However, as the husband, wife, life partner or family member of a person with Dementia, you will most likely feel it is your responsibility and duty to at least be involved in the primary caring role.

You may be still working full time and need your income to support your joint living costs. For a while, working part-time may be possible if you can make alternative arrangements for your role as a primary Dementia carer.

Financial concerns may add to your distress and shock after the diagnosis of Dementia. Working out how to provide the financial support necessary may not be a simple matter for some. For others it may be necessary to sell the family home, in order to provide for future nursing home care for the person with Dementia. Maintaining two residences for one couple is another expense which may never have been contemplated.

Financial advice from your family, family lawyer, social worker or banker may help you to work out how to overcome these issues.

A Dementia diagnosis may be a complete shock and possibly fill you with fear because of the stigma and lack of knowledge concerning this particular disease. You may not know what caring for a Dementia-impacted person really involves on a daily basis.

I certainly had no idea what was required of me when Fulton was first diagnosed. Planning for what lies ahead may be almost impossible because there are so many unknowns with every stage of the Dementia journey.

If you are a paid carer, it is still a very difficult job. But at least you can escape home after a day's work to a 'normal life'.

A family carer on the other hand has no escape, as they may be caring 24 hours a day. Plus they have to endure and grieve daily for the loss of the person they once knew. This can be emotionally confronting.

In addition to these real worries is the uncertainty and lack of knowledge about how long your caring role will last. Different types of Dementia take longer to develop fully than others. I often asked myself, 'How long will I be fulfilling this role? Will it be two years or ten? How long will my health last?'

As a carer you are therefore faced with many unknowns, uncertainties, and unfamiliar paths to tread on your Dementia journey. To some extent, your own life may be in limbo for many months or even years.

I realised that I had to say goodbye to my former life, in conjunction with farewelling my husband. Although Fulton did not pass away for almost three years after the Dementia diagnosis, the person I knew had gradually disappeared much earlier. Caring for a very different Fulton proved harder than I anticipated. I still loved him very much, but the person I had married existed only in my memory. I had to learn to adjust to the person Fulton had become.

Nobody else could help me with this aspect of caring for him. Occasionally, the fog lifted and I saw a fleeting glimpse of the man I had married.

Sadness was my daily shadow, but I worked hard to keep moving forward, and tried to find something to smile about each day. *Smile and the whole world smiles with you, cry and you cry alone ...*

When Blanche and I started to correspond about caring for our husbands, I do not think either of us would have predicted that our tenuous connection would lead to us both learning so much about Dementia. It was a real bonus for me to have a fellow traveller on the Dementia journey.

I am a very private person and did not often share my feelings of frustration, anxiety, sadness and grief with anyone. There are some things no mother wants to share with her children about their father.

After connecting with Blanche over our shared roles as carers of our husbands, I realised Blanche was experiencing the same issues as I was. This made it so much easier for me to open up to her about just how devastated I was by the impact of Dementia on our marriage. She understood!

Soon Blanche and I started to share our daily experiences. The ringing of the phone at night became a welcome sound signalling the chance to share our daily challenges, sometimes over a glass of wine or a cup of tea. And we started to find it possible to laugh at some of the bizarre incidents that had marked that day.

Blanche's difficulties in caring for Jack in the early stages of Dementia (before the formal diagnosis was confirmed by doctors), were similar to mine with Fulton.

However Jack had a definitive diagnosis well before he reached the final stage of the disease. So Blanche had ample time to arrange for him to go into a nursing home, before he had reached the most difficult stage of high care. Also, their doctor did prescribe some medications which provided some support for Jack.

Fulton's diagnosis came much later, when he was well into the mid-stage of Dementia. So Fulton and I had to manage our lives with minimal medical support. This was due not only to a misdiagnosis, but also to the fact that Fulton refused to seek any further medical opinions after he was diagnosed with prostate cancer.

Although Blanche and I shared the commonality of a Dementia diagnosis, our caring pathways and our husbands' caring needs were very different, as yours may be.

Some of this was due to obvious differences in our backgrounds and lifestyles, but I believe the main differences were due to the different timing of the clinical diagnosis.

Jack had been treated by doctors for a couple of years and was diagnosed when he was still in the early stage of Dementia. Fulton on the other hand was not diagnosed until he was well progressed into his Dementia journey. So we had lost precious time when Fulton's brain was only mildly impacted by Dementia. Had we known earlier, we could have ticked off some of the goals on our bucket list, like travelling overseas again. Also, we definitely would have spent more time with our children and grandchildren.

Caring for Fulton at home after his diagnosis presented me with challenges that I had never faced before. I researched online and borrowed every library book on Dementia that I could find. I searched through every bookshop in Canberra and actually spent a fortune buying books on the topic. I watched every documentary and movie with Dementia as the main theme.

I became an expert on Alzheimer's and Dementia, but learned very little about how to best care for or help my husband. Nothing I read really prepared me for the daily challenges I faced trying to help Fulton in the time he spent at home before going into full-time care in a nursing home. I could find nothing published about caring for a person suffering from Dementia.

I did find a wealth of information on the different types of Dementia, the symptoms, the stages from low care to high care, but nothing on how to communicate and care for a high-care person suffering from Dementia. Most of the articles and journals were brimming with information that was academic and scientific in content, rather than practical information on how to care for a person with Dementia. Research and development is an essential part of the Dementia story, but these articles were of little help to me in my efforts to find how I could best care for Fulton.

In reality, my questions were finally answered over time by trial and error. So of course I made lots of mistakes, but so too did I discover useful tools to support me in my caring role for Fulton.

In hindsight, I realise in my research I was looking for only part of what I needed to know.

What I should have been researching was, 'How does a fit and healthy wife, mother, grandmother change her life completely to devote every minute of the day and night to the care for her husband, who has reached the advanced stages of Dementia? How does she renegotiate her relationship with everyone, including her family?'

Family relationships will change as the Dementia progresses and the carer's role becomes a 24/7 job.

As a wife and mother, I had been very independent – but as a carer I needed to learn to become more dependent on medical experts and my children for help in caring for Fulton. This was not easy for anyone especially family members who were used to parents who had been very independent. Fulton's illness impacted us all differently.

Possibly in some families a wife may be expected to be totally responsible for the care of her husband in all ways – emotional, physical and financial. There is no exemplar for how each family works out the way to navigate their Dementia journey.

In discussing this aspect of how to care for a person living with Dementia I am constantly amazed at the diversity of choices made.

It is sad that in some instances the wife may have to bear this burden almost totally single-handed. The reasons for this are many – they may be cultural, or children may be engaged in their own families and careers, or they may just be selfish and believe that it is Mum's job to look after Dad.

There are a number of related groups like the Dementia Association and charitable and church groups which can help in a multitude of ways.

Also, I have found that often adult sons will leave the care of their parent with Dementia to their sisters, wives or partners.

It must be very challenging for unmarried or single Dementia sufferers to try to stay in their own home without close family support. The problems which a single person will face are not insurmountable if they can arrange for their own care in the case of illness whilst they are still healthy and of sound mind.

This is why both 'Power of Attorney' and 'End of Life' care plans should be discussed with either your family, close friends and your family lawyer, when you are in good health.

What I really needed in those early days of caring for Fulton was what Blanche and I are trying to accomplish by sharing our stories and tips with you, as a Dementia carer: a unique and practical guide for the Dementia carer documenting specific behaviours you have to cope with on a daily basis and share with you are lessons learnt by providing you with tips we have learnt along our journeys.

In sharing and documenting some of my experiences with Fulton in my emails with Blanche, I wanted to prepare her for what lay ahead, as I had not been prepared, nor did I have a guide, when I originally commenced our journey. I hoped my anecdotal stories would allow her to develop coping skills, so Blanche could last the journey to the final destination.

I believe my caring role would have been much easier if I had known all that could be involved and I, and the family, would have made some joint preparations.

Forewarned is fore-armed ...

At the time I made endless mistakes due to my total lack of understanding of how to best care for Fulton and myself. The family all rallied around and offered to help us in whatever way they could. However, they all had their own lives, and I did not want to abnegate my duty as a wife and mother.

When requesting help, I never thought to ask the family for respite care for myself so I could have some time just to take care of my needs. I only asked for the family's help if I needed assistance with Fulton, such as taking him to medical appointments, as it was dangerous to drive with him in the car alone.

One of the best things I did, in a practical sense, to make our life easier in those first few months after diagnosis, was to implement a routine which we followed loosely each day.

I even found a whiteboard, which on one side I marked out with our weekly calendar; on the other side was our daily schedule. It was very easy to rub out each week and write in new changes with the marker as they came up. I guess having been a schoolteacher for many years, I found a timetable helped me to use my time most effectively. I could take a quick look at it and work out when I could fit in a hair appointment or a shopping trip when Fulton was out with friends.

Fulton, during his long career, had always used a diary, so for him it was a familiar thing to do. He had always carried his diary with him from appointment to appointment and upgraded it as necessary. Although the format was different to his diary, he was happy to see his day at a glance on the whiteboard sitting on our sideboard.

We could both see the appointments and commitments for the week, so it was easy to fit in a walk or visit to one of our daughters without double-booking a lunch with his mates. When friends rang and wanted to take Fulton to lunch it was easy to see which time was free for the week. Fulton was in the habit of checking the whiteboard as we ate breakfast and saying, 'What are we doing today?'

I organised our daily schedule into activities in the morning when Fulton's brain was working well, to quiet activities and rest in the afternoon when he often became tired, anxious and overwrought.

Introducing the whiteboard was a simplistic thing to do, but reaped such rewards in keeping our life running smoothly that I feel it was one of the most valuable tools I introduced into my caring world.

The other practical thing I did was to have my notebook with me at all times. It was like an old-fashioned address book in diary format listed alphabetically. Tips and advice from doctors, carers and friends were entered regularly. Over time I had filled my notebook with information on nursing homes, lawyers, doctors/specialist appointments and discussions, key medical contacts, prescription details, emergency contacts and other incidental information. I must say it proved invaluable on many occasions to have all this information readily available in one spot. Mobile phones and computers may be your choice, but I found my old notebook irreplaceable.

For a brief period after diagnosis we were able to still go out and enjoy visiting family and friends. I was conscious that Fulton was not at ease and would become anxious and disoriented if I left his side.

One of the last lunches we attended, before declining all invitations, was a charity fundraiser held one Sunday afternoon. Most of the other guests were known to us and our host was one of the few people who knew Fulton had been diagnosed with Dementia. At first I had declined the invitation but our friend persuaded me 'to come along it will do you both good and I will keep an eye on Fulton'.

All went well till after lunch it was announced that dessert, coffee and tea were available at the buffet. I stood up to go to the buffet but our host said quietly to me, 'It's OK, Jenny, sit down and relax. Come on, Fulton, we'll get coffee and tea for the ladies.'

I was apprehensive as I lost sight of Fulton – he disappeared in the crowd for what felt like an eternity.

Trying to disguise my escalating fear from my friends, I scanned the room helplessly looking for him. Finally, I managed to catch sight of him, only to see from across the room, another guest had momentarily distracted our host who was accompanying him, leaving Fulton alone.

Fulton quickly disappeared from my view into the crowd milling around the buffet table. My heart initially sank, thoughts racing. I started to think of excuses to leave the guests seated around me, in order to seek Fulton out and ensure he was safe and hadn't escaped down the street!

Just at that moment Fulton reappeared. Relieved, I motioned for him to rejoin me at my side, however he returned to the table with his coffee in one hand, and placed a saucer holding a limp wet tea bag in front of me! 'There's your tea, darling,' he said and pulled his chair out, misjudged the distance, and promptly sat on the floor with a loud thud!

Of course, the other guests at the table were perplexed by his behaviour and I heard murmurs of 'Poor Fulton'. I hoped they had not assumed he had consumed too much red wine! I was embarrassed for him, but Fulton seemed totally unaware of what he had done. After he had been helped back up onto his chair, he looked over at the tea bag I had not touched and said, 'Didn't you want tea?'

In the car on the way home, Fulton was restless and agitated but did not mention the incident. The next few days at home were a bit of a nightmare as he became increasingly restless, agitated and short-tempered.

Nothing like that had ever happened before, but I realised Fulton's condition was escalating. As his carer I decided then that I would not place him in situations again which, were now challenging and beyond his capabilities.

Shortly afterwards, when I related this episode to his neurologist, she confirmed it was best not to place Fulton in situations which could cause his Dementia behaviours to escalate.

However until something like this happens, it is hard to judge or identify what situations or circumstances will cause the person you are caring for to escalate into this type of Dementia behaviour. I did however, notice that his spatial awareness appeared 'off'. Simple tasks like going to sit down or stand up, reaching for a door knob, getting in and out of the car, or taking stairs could result in him stumbling or falling.

Whilst there are some household or mobility aides, such as bed hoists, walking canes or swivel seats for example, they might not be suitable for you and the Dementia person you are caring for. I did try a few of these ideas. Some were disastrous failures – and some Fulton just simply threw out or hid!

So I decided not to take Fulton out anymore where he did not feel safe. I felt it best just to keep our social activities restricted to our own home environment and only invited a couple of close friends who would not be worried by Fulton's unusual and sometimes bizarre behaviours.
The unpredictability of Fulton's behaviour became one of the hardest tasks for me to cope with on a daily basis, as his carer and as his wife.

I found friends were varied in their response to Fulton's illness. Just as I was unsure of what to do, so too were they. I had no ill feeling to their lack of support, as I think it was hard for them to know what to do to help, or even what to say.

Some, like Sara and Athol, were very supportive, joining us regularly for a glass of wine or a coffee on a Sunday afternoon.

Athol even visited Fulton when I was interstate and Fulton was in a respite care facility. I really appreciated their company and support, but after a few months I had to stop inviting them home as Fulton became agitated and annoyed with himself, as he could no longer cope with simple conversation, which frustrated him greatly.

He was embarrassed that he could not play host by pouring a glass of wine for our guests. Yet he hated seeing anyone else do the things he had always done and was angry as he really did not understand what had happened to prevent him from carrying out these simple tasks. His annoyance at himself was sometimes vocalised in anger, 'Bloody hell, what am I to do?' or by walking away and refusing to sit and relax and join our guests. I tried to calm him down as we all just wanted him to be happy and enjoy our time together.

His close friends Bill and Bruce stood by us throughout his illness, and in fact Bill visited him on the day he passed away. Other friends and business colleagues fell by the wayside, and apart from a few phone calls to check on his health, I did not see them again until his funeral. Although I was upset at so many people drifting away from us, I understood completely as there is a stigma about Dementia and it seemed some friends did not know how to help, what to do, or what to say. I found this quite hurtful, but I did not have the time to worry too much about being ostracised by some when they finally learned of Fulton's illness.

A recent survey in Australia of nearly 6,000 people with Dementia and their carers found 71% had not been included in family activities, while 80% had experienced people going out of their way to avoid a friend or relative with Dementia. (Sydney's *Daily Telegraph*, 21 September 2020, page 9).

In the early days, I should probably have asked for more help just for myself, as I really did not know the extent of the emotional and physical toll the caring role was having on me or would have in the future. Some friends and family just do not know what to say or do.

I remember on one occasion I arranged to meet Fiona for a quick coffee during her lunch hour. As she sat down, she handed me a huge bunch of flowers and I dissolved into floods of tears. I am not overly emotional and certainly not prone to tears, but her gesture just overwhelmed me.

She did not need to say anything, but I knew she understood how her father's illness was impacting me. I would drag myself out of bed every morning thinking that I did not know how I would get through the day. I remember one of the children saying reproachfully to me one day, 'Why do you leave me alone with Dad every time I visit?'

I had not realised I was doing this. Well, the truth was that maybe I needed to have some time alone. Due to Fulton's escalating Dementia behaviours, spending day after day with him was a difficult thing to do. By this time, there was no logical or conventional conversation possible. All I could do was to provide him with a comfortable and loving, caring environment. But we were both locked in, like prisoners in solitary confinement. I found our enforced isolation together hard to deal with at times. So I guess I took advantage of the opportunity to escape occasionally when one of the children visited.

Sometimes, I would sit for a while with whichever of the children was visiting and say, 'I hope you don't mind if I pop out to do some shopping', or 'I just need to do some vacuuming upstairs', or whatever came into my mind!

Perhaps I gave the impression that I was not interested in seeing them, which was of course far from how I felt.

With the knowledge I now have, it would have been much better for everyone if we had collaborated more on setting up a family schedule for minding Fulton and giving me a break on a regular basis.

I did not realise at the time these visits were quite traumatic for the children, as it was hard for them to witness the continuing deterioration of their father. Losing a parent is never easy, but losing a person who is physically present, but mentally absent, is a burden which is difficult to cope with. It was difficult for us all to understand that visiting Mum and Dad was totally different now Dad had Dementia. The children and I took a long time to realise everything had changed, not just Dad.

In my new role as a carer I had to learn appropriate ways to communicate with Fulton. Having been married for 40 years, we had learned to communicate well on every level. We had a great relationship built on mutual love and trust. We had no secrets from each other. We conversed about anything and everything.

Given the nature of his work, he had met so many interesting people and visited and lived in so many exiting places. Life with Fulton was never boring. The best thing was we both had a good sense of humour.

Sadly, now there really was no interesting conversation between us, only the sound of my voice. Now his vocabulary was limited to only a few words. He was able occasionally to show flashes of his fast wit and clever mind. Sometimes the fog would lift, and I would see glimpses of the person he had once been. Sadly, he knew that he was changing and that annoyed him and he became frustrated at not understanding the simplest conversation or being able to express his needs and wants.

A couple of times he grabbed my hand and said, 'I'm sorry, darling, to do this to us.' That broke my heart as none of what we were going through was his fault. But how could I explain this to him? He no longer understood much of what I, or anyone else, said.

Usually when a partner is struck with a life-threatening or life-changing illness, the couple can share their burden of fear, loss and grief together. They will have the chance to reminisce over their shared memories, the joys and sorrows of family life.

The rites of passage of their children, the graduation ceremonies, overseas trips, the birth of their first grandchildren.

Dementia, even in the early stages, took this away – as I found there could not be any conversation of this nature. However I did keep trying to communicate with him, right until the day he died, that I was happy to have the chance to be with him and help him on this journey. I certainly felt pleased that I had the health and resilience to keep Fulton at home for as long as I did. Later I grieved for him, but also for our shared old age, which prior to his Dementia diagnosis we had both been looking forward to, after raising our children. Time together was to be our special wish. Ironically, as it turned out, we had time alone but not the way we had planned.

When he could no longer easily find his way around our home. Fiona and Alycia made a number of identifiable labels for the cupboard doors, fridge, bathroom, front door and so on. Soon the whiteboard became redundant for Fulton as he could no longer read – but I kept it on the sideboard so the carers could check what was on the day's schedule.

In time he started to regularly escape into the front garden many times a day looking for the way upstairs to his bedroom, and would become annoyed to find he was unexpectedly outside our home. Then he would have no idea where he was or how he got there. He was constantly lost in every way possible – physically, emotionally and mentally. He would then become agitated, annoyed and fearful, and would hurriedly leave our home and walk quickly out the gate and rush up the road as fast as he could. It seemed to me this wish to escape from home was the only way he felt he could escape from Dementia. So the signs the girls made were helpful at first, for a short time when he could still read. After a while we drew identifying pictures like a preschool has for its non-verbal children.

Eventually, Fulton lost all sense of where he was, and had to be taken everywhere by hand. He was no longer able to converse about a range of topics but could respond to simple questions such as, 'Do you want a coffee?' or 'Are you hungry?'

As his cognitive ability deteriorated and was diminished by the plaque overtaking his brain, it was pointless to reason with him that some of his behaviour had become unacceptable.

Not only this, but he became an expert escapologist who could have put Houdini to shame. He was like quicksilver escaping from our home when I was momentarily distracted by a phone call or our little dog Edith wanting some attention.

As soon as my back was turned he could disappear. Wandering off quickly is a characteristic shared by toddlers and some people having Dementia.

It is good to be prepared for this possibility by ensuring the person you are caring for has full self-identification containing their name, address, medical details and of course your contact information, in a pocket or wallet to be kept on their person at all times.

Fortunately, there is now a watch available specifically for seniors which has GPS installed.

Sadly for me I had not followed my own advice earlier in my caring journey and my family and I spent many heart-stopping hours searching the local suburb looking for Fulton. His refusal to return home on these episodes could be scary, embarrassing and challenging. If I managed to grab his arm, he would sometimes pull away like a child not wanting to go to school.

One afternoon when he went missing from home on one of his wanderings, I found it so hard to explain to a neighbour, watering his garden as we ran past, why I was pleading for Fulton to 'please come back home with me'.

On this part of our journey, when all else failed, I used a method of trial and error to see what worked best to defuse the particular behaviour on the day that was causing a problem. Plus I had a locksmith install the type of locking devices used on nursing home doors, which rang loudly if the door was opened! This helped a great deal when he crept quietly out of the home in the early hours of the morning, whilst I was sleeping.

So I learned to use different methods of distraction as each Dementia behaviour appeared. This was the only way I could try to keep our daily interactions as calm and pleasant as possible.

Life for me became a rollercoaster. One day Fulton would be almost his former persona – kind, considerate, loving and of course charming. Then suddenly a switch would go in his brain, and he would become a raging, furiously angry person behaving like a toddler, having a temper tantrum for seemingly no reason. It was never easy to distract him when he was off on one of these 'dummy spits'.

On these occasions I found TV was my saviour. I had taped hours of his favourite shows like *Yes, Minister*, *Keeping Up Appearances* and his two favourite movies *The Great Escape* and *Lawrence of Arabia*. These were long-time favourites of his.

The movies were great as they both ran over two hours! I would sit with him on the sofa for twenty minutes or so until he was fully absorbed, before I left him to start on my regular household chores. Sometimes after the movie started, I could even pop up to the shops to grab a few things. The best thing about Fulton watching these movies is that he could never remember the ending so was happy to watch them over and over again! I could relax knowing he would not be upset by, or even notice, my absence. When I returned home a half an hour later, he would be sitting contentedly watching Steve McQueen's escape from his prisoner of war camp, along with other men captured by the Germans during World War Two. Often he would have fallen asleep.

Ironically, later as the Dementia progressed, I regretted this choice of film when he kept trying to escape from his nursing home and tried to involve other patients in his plans!

When I had an appointment nearby, I would put his favourite cheese and ham sandwiches, a slice of fruit cake and a thermos of coffee on a tray and place it on a table within

Fulton's reach. He was happy to have his favourite movie to watch along with his favourite food to snack on. He had long since lost the ability to prepare himself simple food like a piece of toast. He could no longer find a cup or plate or turn on a kettle to boil water. So after preparing food for him to be consumed as he watched his favourite TV shows I quietly left the house. Often, he did not even notice my absence but thought I was probably working in another room upstairs. By this stage he was unable to open the front door, so I no longer had the worry of him escaping.

These arrangements were important for me because it enabled me to have some time to do the shopping alone. After losing Fulton on a few occasions, I had learned the hard way not to take him to the shopping mall. All carers need to work out a plan that works in their own particular caring scenario.

Establishing some type of schedule early in the caring journey makes it much easier than trying to establish a routine when the person with Dementia can no longer understand simple tasks or requests.

When Fulton was in the early stages of Dementia we always shopped together however, after he disappeared a few times in the mall, I found it better to leave him at home watching his favourite television show.

Music also calmed him down if he was having a bad day, but it had to be the right music to suit the mood of the day. Fulton loved any type of classical music, and I made several tapes of his favourites which I played for hours every day. Music kept him calm.

A regular trigger for his 'dummy spits' was the phone ringing, disturbing his viewing and frightening him. He could not distinguish between the TV remote, the landline phone and my mobile. So if the phone rang when he was watching TV, he would grab the remote, always tightly clutched in his hand, and place it to his ear, 'Hello, who is it?'

Of course the phone would keep ringing until I picked up. Fulton would be yelling his greeting more frequently into the remote, and commenced to shout at the remote loudly becoming more and more agitated and angry if the phone continued to ring. Meantime, I was trying to speak calmly to the person at the end of the phone. This happened numerous times until I had to disconnect our landline and make sure my mobile was on vibrate or silent in my pocket or hanging around my neck, in other words, nowhere near Fulton.

Any sudden noise like the phone or the doorbell ringing sent him into a panic reaction which, caused him to try to move or run away from the sound.

In the beginning of these outbursts I tried to explain to Fulton that he was holding a TV remote and the phone was on the kitchen bench, but he just did not and could not understand that. Eventually during one his episodes, he pulled the landline cord off the wall, smashing the phone to smithereens and creating a huge hole in the wall. I just put a chair in front of the hole, and had it fixed a few years later.

A close friend of Fulton's commented to me at that time how frustrating it was that we no longer had a landline!
I wanted to scream at him, 'If only you knew why we don't have a landline.' I just stopped myself from giving him the full brunt of my pent-up frustration.

Frustration! Exasperation! Irritation!

I thought, 'You cannot even come close to understanding how frustrating it can be to care for someone with Dementia.'

But being a polite and calm person, through gritted teeth and a forced smile, I replied sweetly, 'I am sorry you feel like that but you can text or call me anytime on my mobile or email me whenever you wish.' Needless to say we did not hear from him again.

I found sometimes I needed another method to distract Fulton. To stop his tantrums, I learned to quickly turn the phone off and suggest we take Edith for a walk. Distraction worked best when trying to defuse a tantrum. I learned that trying to use a logical explanation would only escalate his anger or confusion.

On these walks, which were frequent – Edith had never been taken for so many walks prior to Fulton's Dementia diagnosis – just being away from our home relaxed us both. Canberra is referred to as the 'Bush Capital', so we were spoilt for choice when it comes to choosing parks or walkways to meander through.

As the Dementia progressed, I found Fulton started to develop a peculiar physical trait, he appeared to lose the ability to properly lift or raise his feet and legs when he walked, so he appeared to shuffle, rather than walk. This dragging of his feet could easily cause him to stumble. It was no good giving him a walking stick, as I had tried to. Somehow he managed to get it caught between his legs. To my horror, on another occasion he attempted to use it as a weapon, when a young dog ran to greet us.

So he tended to lean on me quite heavily to aid his balance. As we slowly made our way along the suburban roads near our home, I felt we resembled a small yacht listing to one side on a windless sea. I thought a puff of wind would have easily knocked us both over.

Fulton had a number of falls in our home at this time, so I held his arm firmly to avoid any more accidents. We did not talk much on these walks but were both content to wander along taking in the beauty of the local suburban gardens as if they were the Tuileries Gardens in Paris. I loved escaping from our home almost as much as Fulton did, as home was fast becoming our prison.

Sometimes we would walk to our local bakery – a croissant and a hot coffee would mend our broken souls and lift our spirits – as if we were both escaping back into 'normal life', for a moment. Things that we both may have taken for granted in the past – like enjoying the sights, sounds and 'people-watching' at our local cafe – I now would relish as quiet shared moments together.

Those of us who have lived with the sadness and unpredictability of the Dementia journey can appreciate just how the banality of a small local shopping precinct can bring so much pleasure. Children skipping past us, the local greenie riding up and parking her bike, the young mum pushing her baby to do her shopping, all added to our wellbeing.

Previously our shared joy in participating in a range of enjoyable activities and socialising with friends over a lovely long meal with lots of wine and interesting repartee, were no longer possible.

Fulton was not aware of our lost world, but I was reminded every day. So I savoured the little that we could now do together. The bakery staff knew us well and were so kind to Fulton. I bought the newspapers and we often passed a pleasant hour reading the papers and sipping our coffee. By this stage Fulton could no longer actually read, but enjoyed what had been a familiar routine. Frequently, his paper was upside-down but the good thing was that it was a shared activity we could still both enjoy. He insisted on paying for these escapades and would nonchalantly hand over a $50 bill, for a $10 charge and say, 'Keep the change!' The waitress would diplomatically slip me the change when Fulton was momentarily distracted.

You may wonder why Fulton had a $50 note with him. Well, that is another story. Fulton could not remember our address, the suburb in which we lived or our phone number. So in the early days after diagnosis, when he was still able to socialise with friends, he would meet them at the university for lunch about once a week. Continuing these long-time activities was very important for Fulton, but also enabled his friends to interact with him whilst he was still able to communicate with them.

Usually I drove him to these lunches, and after lunch his friends would arrange for our usual cabby, George the taxi driver, to collect him. Fulton's friends would phone me to let me know he was on his way home. The taxi fare was around $45. This arrangement meant Fulton kept a little independence, and I was able to use the two hours he was away to catch up with household chores, go shopping and attend medical appointments or just potter at home. I had made a little card for Fulton to show the taxi driver, which contained all his address details. This stayed in his suit pocket along with a $50 note in his wallet, to pay the driver.

This was reassuring to us both, until the day he unknowingly dropped the card as he got into the taxi. It was a new driver who did not know where he lived! Fulton's friend had given directions to the driver however. Apparently he remembered the suburb but had forgotten the street name and number.

When Fulton was unable to tell him his address, he told the driver to drop him off at our local shops, a place that was very familiar due to our daily walks. Sadly, he became disoriented and lost, which resulted in him randomly walking around the surrounding suburbs for a couple of hours in the wrong direction before, thankfully, I found him totally exhausted, fearful and anxious.

That was his last trip alone, but I made sure he always had the $50 in his wallet plus 3 cards containing his details and headed 'In case of emergency, please contact etc'.

In addition I wrote the sentence, 'The bearer of this card has Dementia.' The latter piece of information came in handy on a number of occasions, when I could show it to an anxious person who was concerned or confused by Fulton's behaviour.

I remember Blanche telling me she found this card useful when she was travelling in Italy with Jack. When checking in at the airport, Jack had an incident and Blanche was able to explain quietly to the immigration officer what the problem was, by showing her the card.

I also used the card on several occasions, rather than saying 'My husband has Dementia', which I felt may embarrass Fulton and I wanted to try to preserve his dignity. I believe this card would also be useful should Fulton become lost again.

The difficulties of driving with Fulton as a passenger in the car increased over time – particularly when he reached what would become the 'final stage' of Dementia – to the point where he became dangerous. Then I found driving with Fulton was akin to riding shotgun on a Cobb&Co stagecoach in the early days of settlement. I had to be on full alert for a sudden attack at any time, not from bushrangers, but from my dearly beloved seated beside me.

The trouble was I was driving along highways in heavy traffic at speeds of 80km an hour.

An attack from the side, when Fulton grabbed the gear stick, pulled my hair, or tried to open the car door in his attempt to escape and 'commando roll' from the car, could have had terrible repercussions.

I know he was not truly cognisant or aware of the danger he was putting us both into when he would behave this way. My children had previously raised their concerns with me but now they were increasingly concerned about Fulton's behaviours in the car. His unpredictable behaviours in the car and mood swings had become more frequent and volatile.

Soon all the activities arranged by the Alzheimer's Association for people having Dementia, and the trips to visit the family and medical appointments, became an impossibility for me to do alone. Using a taxi was an alternative that worked for a while, as I could sit beside Fulton on the back seat and distract him from his interest in opening the door while we were driving. When essential, I used a hire car service along with a family member who could take time off work, so the two of us could sit either side of Fulton to keep him from doing anything dangerous. Soon that too became too difficult to manage and we became totally housebound, except for an occasional walk on a day when Fulton was relaxed.

We were both very private people and had always valued our privacy. This was probably one of the reasons we lived in the country on our farm, our nearest neighbours being a few kilometres away from our home. Paradoxically, we loved socialising and meeting people, but our own home was sacrosanct. I therefore resisted having carers come into our home to help take care of Fulton for as long as possible. Also I believed, as his wife, it was my job to care for him.

However, after several months of challenging episodes and experiencing numerous scary events during the night, when he screamed or called out loudly, convinced wild dogs were tearing him apart, I realised we needed help.

The doctor told me these hallucinations were part of having Dementia but offered no medication or advice, except to advise me to put Fulton into a nursing home. I believe a mild sleeping tablet could have helped, but I toughed it out, without Fulton ever being offered any calming medication.

My problem was that I was getting very little sleep because of Fulton's night terrors. I was becoming physically exhausted in my full-time caring role. My sleep was broken every night by Fulton's terrifying nightmares when he tossed and turned, sometimes grabbing me in a frightening grasp. Sometimes he would fall out of bed during one of these nightmares, and I would spend ages trying to lift him back into the bed. He would stay asleep so he was a dead weight. It was frightening to me, but at that time I did not tell family members about these events, as I did not want to burden them with something else that could not be fixed.
Many nights I had no sleep at all.

Eventually, I moved into another bedroom and placed a bell on his door to alert me if he was out of bed. Even so, I still got up to check on him several times a night. It was just as I had done when our children were babies. Looking after a baby however, does bring joy.

I just felt inadequate during this part of my caring role. I knew now I would have to place Fulton in full-time care, but I resisted making a final decision. My children were worried about my health and safety. They all helped me as much as they possibly could. I was aware they were not only grieving for the father they were losing, but were worried about me. I had recently had a hip replacement and a fall could have caused major problems for me.

It was just as I had reached near total exhaustion that I knew it was time to arrange for help in the home.

Dressing Fulton and helping with his morning rituals became extremely difficult. I always hung up his clothes each night in preparation for the following day to save time. Trying to help him with showering also was a bit of a nightmare as usually I was soaked while trying to physically move him out of the shower.

Now simple daily tasks were like competing in a marathon. After hesitating for a few months, I finally made the decision to arrange for carers to come and help me look after Fulton for a couple of hours each day. I was worried about his reaction as he had adamantly refused to have help in the home early after diagnosis. I reluctantly came to the realisation that due to his Dementia needs, my role as his Dementia carer had reached capacity, and having a carer in the home was now not a choice. Rather, now it had become what both Fulton and I needed.

It was the best decision for us, as I found his daily carers were just amazing. They were professional, kind, thorough and knew just how to approach Fulton so that he felt safe. He was so vulnerable and, just like a toddler, he was scared of strangers.

Over a couple of weeks, I introduced them to Fulton one by one. And although he had never liked having strangers care for him, he gradually permitted them to help me undress and shower him. A week or so later when they had won his confidence. I was able to withdraw and let them do these tasks alone.

It was so good to be able to get him into bed at a normal time. Prior to having carers, Fulton would tell me he was not tired and would refuse to go to bed. I could not leave him alone downstairs, as he might wander outside trying to find the way to our bedroom. Consequently, I often sat up with him past midnight or later to be sure he was safe. Of course, because he did very little except eat and sleep all day, he did not tire as quickly as I did at night.

Getting Fulton into bed sounds easy, but he had no concept of how to move from a standing to a sitting position on the side of the bed, to turning and placing his head on the pillow whilst lifting his legs onto the bed. I had to climb behind him on the bed and help him to turn his upper body around while I tried to lift his legs from the floor onto the bed. This manoeuvre required the skills of an Olympic gymnast or Yoga enthusiast! Many times we both ended up in a heap, laughing, with Fulton lying sideways on our bed whilst I tried to move his legs up off the floor.

Putting a Dementia patient to bed as a carer certainly requires skill, strength and patience. It was sad to experience Fulton's loss of his athletic ability, especially since as a young man he had been a keen sportsman and had played rugby, tennis and golf for many years. Now he could not get into bed unaided. Dementia can be cruel.

Establishing a bedtime routine was just as hard as it had been when the children were toddlers. Sometimes I resorted to turning the television off and telling Fulton the station had closed for the night. He would then still tell me he wanted to stay up longer, just like a defiant child would sit staring at the blank screen.

However everything changed when the carers arrived. He had always had great respect for anyone in a uniform, especially nurses as he felt they did a wonderful service to the community.

During the evening bedtime routine, Fulton became quite compliant to the carer's gentle request, 'Come on, Fulton, time for bed.'

I stayed downstairs while the carer helped Fulton into his pyjamas, bathed, cleaned teeth and helped him into bed. Once that ritual was over and she said goodnight to Fulton, I would retreat upstairs to watch the news with him. He was relaxed and always fell asleep quickly.

I think he had finally agreed to the carers helping him, as I recently had hip surgery and he knew bending and lifting him into bed was painful for me.

Our carers came twice a day morning and evening to shower and dress Fulton. It usually took about an hour at each session. I not only enjoyed their real skill in handling Fulton's needs, but also I enjoyed the cups of tea and chats we often had before they left us for another job. Their knowledge of Dementia was invaluable, and for the first time I was able to talk to somebody who had an intimate experience of caring for a person with Dementia. I learned about the disease, and what to expect as Fulton's condition escalated. They imparted their 'lived Dementia carer' experience, wisdom and information which, I had not found in any of the books I had read.

After several months the different carers all expressed the observation that I should perhaps consider putting Fulton into a nursing home. They could see he was deteriorating and that I was finding it difficult to manage his needs, day and night. At this stage, a carer came in for an hour every morning and night, seven days a week to take care of Fulton's personal care.

Then on Fridays, another carer came to take Fulton for an outing during the day. At first he refused to move and sat sullenly with his arms folded on the lounge. But when a different young woman turned up, everything changed. She had a happy disposition and managed to engage Fulton by chatting about her love of basketball. She was very tall and they looked an odd couple as they set off in her little car to go to the War Memorial, Art Gallery or just for a walk. Fulton grew to love these trips and told me he was glad to be able to teach his new carer as, 'She knows nothing about anything!'

She later told me she really enjoyed these outings as, 'Fulton knows so much!'

I know Jack too had refused to have carers in the home, but by being patient I had been able to change Fulton's resolve. I was pleased to be able to surrender some of his caring tasks to the professional carers. In the long run it was through receiving their assistance that I was able to keep Fulton at home for so long.

I also found help in an unexpected place: our local pharmacy proved to be a real godsend. Harry our local pharmacist and his staff at Capital Chemist always had a smile and a chat with Fulton.

They tolerated his unusual or unruly behaviour in the shop as he wandered around while I was arranging for his medication to be put into a Webster pack. Although it cost more to have the Webster pack made up, it saved me so much in terms of my time and worry. It was certainly worth the cost involved.

What a wonderful time-saver it was as I just did not have the time to count out Fulton's medication every day. If he was watching me, he would try to grab the tablets I was counting, and attempt to shovel them all into his mouth at once!

An additional bonus with having a friendly pharmacist to whom I could phone through my requests and arrange for another family member to pick up the medication for me. This was such a help when Fulton's behaviour deteriorated, and I could no longer take him for a walk up to our local shops.

At times I was unable to drive Fulton to the doctor to obtain another prescription, and Harry was able to arrange this for me. It sounds like such a small thing to arrange but it was, on occasions, a life-saver for me.

I realised the time was fast approaching when I would have to place Fulton in full-time care. Something which I did not want to do, but finally I had no choice. Keeping Fulton at home became an impossibility as I just could not stay alert and awake 24 hours a day, plus I was finding his increasing tantrums very hard to deal with. Also, it is essential to be well rested to be a good carer, an impossibility if you are being woken up several times a night to take care of a person who hallucinates and falls out of bed. So sadly our next journey was about to begin, which was Fulton's final journey – from our home to the nursing home.

I was fortunate in that I was helped in making the decision to place Fulton in care. He was staying in a respite care facility for a few days, so I could accompany Alycia on a research trip to Victoria. Fulton had expressed his concern at her travelling alone to a remote area to do her work. I suggested we could both go with her, but Fulton said he did not feel up to such a car trip and that I should go with Alycia and he would stay at home. I knew I could not leave him alone as he now was unable to prepare a meal or even to find his way around.

Fortunately, for once, he agreed to go and stay in a respite care facility with no arguments. He had stayed there once before and felt safe there.

I was really pleased for Alycia and myself that we were able to do this trip. We had fun driving there. I enjoyed having normal mother–daughter time, and she had booked us into a beautiful historic hotel on our first night. I think Alycia had wanted to give me a mini-break from my caring duties.

Unfortunately, I received a phone call on the following morning, from the nurse in charge of the respite facility asking me to return immediately to take Fulton home, as he had created 'problems' all night for the other patients and nurses alike. She told me that Fulton should be in full-time care. From her experiences with him, she felt there was no way that I could safely care for him alone any longer.

Alycia and I drove back to Canberra immediately so I could make the necessary arrangements. In many ways I was pleased this decision had been made for me by a health care professional. I had wondered how long I could keep caring for Fulton at home, especially as I was only just surviving on a couple of hours of interrupted sleep every night.

So now the next part of our Dementia journey began.

BLANCHE AND JACK'S STORY

Dear Jenny
At least you had the sound of eggshells. For Jack and me it was a solitary experience, with Jack withdrawing into his thoughts and I was left in isolation with my doubts, pitched in a whirlpool of anxiety, with no real answers and reaching a fevered point with no solutions ...

***

I clearly remember, as if it happened yesterday, coming home with my first-born child and laying her down and saying, 'What am I to do with you?'

Yet I had nine months to plan for my mother-care role and had made a conscious choice to be a 'mother'! However, when I held my child, I still felt my tummy tighten, knowing I was untrained and unprepared to take on this mother-care role, without past experience.

Strangely I felt the same again, after I received the Dementia diagnosis. Acute fear gripped me, as I already had small glimpses of an altered marital relationship. Noticeable too was the financial strain. Our quality of life began to change, with acute isolation and the missed social opportunities that were part-and-parcel of the carer role.

I did not make the choice to be my husband's carer, but I was thrust into taking on this care role, and had to share the journey with Jack, because he was unfortunate to get touched by the disease. Particularly harrowing was the experience after the diagnosis is delivered. There was no immediate interventional advice, as the consulting timeframe does not allow you to access support at such visits. We had to wait for weeks, first to see the GP, and then there was a clear process to follow, managed by a team of neurological medical experts.

Besides, family and friends were unwilling to come forward with help, because in many instances people are uncomfortable to start a Dementia conversation even though Dementia is common in our community. Generally if a person is not personally touched by the disease, then most people know of someone who has been touched, yet there is not enough Dementia-related conversation happening, when compared to other diseases.

Interestingly, both the care roles I have experienced were of a caregiving nature and yet they are vastly different.

My care role when I raised my children was filled with countless moments of immense joy and endless job satisfaction to see the little ones grow, learn and become independent and move forward each day.

Caring for a person living with Dementia is the reverse. I did not start my relationship with Jack as his carer. He was a fiercely independent person, and now as his carer, I found myself acting as his 'enabler' as he was already showing limited signs of accessing the necessary services that would enable him to remain independent, both socially and at home.

On my part, the adjustment to take on this role took time. The dependent Jack started to encroach on my time and for a large part of the day my time was taken, immersed in daily care activities to meet his changing needs. I was unable to cope with these sudden changes in our 'new' evolving relationship. I found Jack always nearby, so I could step in when he appeared muddled or stressed, especially in a crowded environment.

When I took on the mother's care role, it was the community nurse who came to my aid, and who shared professional expertise on mother-and-child caring.

Strangely, I found myself again turning to the community service groups, and found support from a team of Dementia experts, who were ever ready to provide guidance to new carers. I slowly gained Dementia awareness which in time allowed me to dispel the acute fear, stress and the uncertainty that this disease throws out to carers.

So far, science has not yet discovered why the brain cells get destroyed and sometimes the prescribed drugs that are administered have been shown to be of little benefit in the long run. The difficulty of care in the early stages is largely the result of the person living with Dementia and their carer not receiving the same level of medical support that is rightfully available and provided to cancer and heart patients when a diagnosis is made.

My reaction to the Dementia diagnosis was overwhelming and it brought mixed feelings. Firstly, although we were both somewhat prepared, nothing can really prepare you to accept the Dementia diagnosis. Secondly, I had to learn how to accept my carer's role and learn ways to cope with the new lifestyle that Jack and I found ourselves experiencing. Love is key here. It would have been unimaginable to care for Jack, had we not experienced a happy and shared past.

Jack, on hearing the confirmation of his diagnosis, decided to remain in an unwelcome silence of fear, and shut himself with his thoughts for several days. Days later he said, 'I know my silence is deafening, but I need to be alone with my thoughts, whilst I still can contemplate my eminent fate. And I am unwilling to share my daily struggles, that in the past I would have accomplished effortlessly.'

Jack's Dementia-impacted brain took years for others to notice. Gradually his decline into forgetfulness, confusion and helplessness was taking shape. It is our brain that sends messages and Jack's brain demonstrated clearly, that it had become faulty and was not doing its job.

In the beginning I had put these symptoms down to a normal part of the ageing process, but Jack experienced acute communication difficulties and an inability to understand people and it was the same for people who came to converse with him. Gradually the communication loss eroded his confidence to make social contact. He became paranoid that his brain was constantly letting him down more often than he liked in the early days.

His memory failure led to immense frustration for us both. Jack severely felt the loss of his memory, yet he knew that he was powerless to stop the erosion! Simple tasks like going to the corner shop or the pharmacy became a stress. He was fully aware of his loss of ability to speak or process speech when he was addressed, and in frustration he would give up and expect me to take over. These were all simple daily activities that previously he would have had no issues in undertaking.

Worse though, was that it became a strain on our relationship!

Prior to the Dementia diagnosis Jack would be on show and would monopolise the social conversation. But the Dementia symptoms put an end to this personality. He would often became restless and would distance himself socially. Sometimes, if he had to face a minor problem, it would stress him out as he just did not know what to do or have the means to handle the problem. Or if someone spoke to him, he was unable to make sense of their words.

Now, reflecting on Jack's changed social behaviours, it was his language difficulties that restrained his socialising. English was also Jack's second language and he had difficulty expressing his pain or discomfort, particularly when he was in an unfamiliar surrounds. This led to emotional behaviour challenges and sometimes a nightmare that I as his carer had to endure! His behaviours would manifest as agitation or social disharmony, and after such social events he would display extreme fatigue, due to the energy he had expended. I later learnt, from friends and family, that he came across as being uninterested in engaging.

However as his carer, I noticed as his condition progressed, so did my despair. Simple tasks of grooming took an inordinate time to complete with his weakened dexterity, and the need for daily assistance. Jack followed the experts' advice of eating better and socialising more, but still his symptoms got progressively worse and his frustrations only amplified!

Yet my mind would not be silent and I prepared a list of questions, for our next visit to the memory clinic:

- What did the diagnosis actually mean?
- Where to from here?
- Why was there no obvious pain or discomfort?
- When does the brain stop functioning?
- How does one cope with personal, physical and emotional needs?

Jack was a spiritual man. He had spent several years travelling around the world observing different religions, and he applied these principles to his way of life, which later became his totem of beliefs.

It pained him to depend on others to meet his care needs, and if he had lived in a country that had jurisdiction to legalise voluntary assisted dying he would front up. In 2020 the Dutch court approved euthanasia in cases of advanced Dementia.

Doctors in the Netherlands are now able to carry out euthanasia on patients with severe Dementia without fear of prosecution, even if the patient did not express a wish to die. This decision followed a landmark case, where a doctor was acquitted of wrongdoing for euthanising a woman with severe Alzheimer's in 2016. This woman however did request the procedure before her memory condition deteriorated.

By contrast, in Australia, our experience with the medical profession showed that medical experts saw Jack's progressive forgetfulness as just one more case which they were addressing. In time the medical team would see thousands more, without early intervention treatments.

The Dementia diagnosis meant death was foreseeable but it takes a long time before a Dementia-impacted person suffers any discomfort or even looks ill. Our family spent years witnessing Jack's progressive loss and he hated this feeling of helplessness.

Life after the Dementia diagnosis had become a journey and I had to allocate time to learn, research and to be constantly organised – like new parents of a toddler. I had to safeguard our home, as Jack was constantly on the move and he needed to be watched.

The interior of our home had to be rearranged to meet Jack's poor balance, erect handrails in the bathroom and stairs, minimise the furniture and remove rugs to avoid falls. Installed automatic exterior lighting, and new locks to avoid wandering, sometimes people living with Dementia can wander in the middle of the night. I had to turn off the gas at the mains after cooking, as Jack started using our electric kettle on the stove, that later I installed a time monitors on many of our electrical gadgets.

I sometimes wondered where my reliable husband had gone. In time the equality in our shared relationship had become one-sided and, in order to cope, I had to organise paid help – as no carer can do it all!

Administration duties were on the increase and so was the financial cost of living. With extra medical visits, pharmacy costs, home and garden maintenance, fees for day care and a plan for the occasional respite care services, I found the extra costs had skyrocketed as Jack was no longer able to share in the household tasks.

Despite Jack's excellent skills to forecast a financial plan for our future, he did not envisage the extra expenses that a carer incurred over the period if one of us had a life-threatening illness and one of us had to live separately. The uncertainty of the illness and the additional expenses all became another added burden on our fixed household budget.

Without doubt, the structured programs led by qualified Dementia professionals and funded by the local council for new carers after the diagnosis supported my coping mechanisms. Learning activities were the key to get many carers informed and to ease carers' stress by directing them to resources and access support services that were on offer in the community.

These new friends were all Dementia carers themselves and experiencing similar challenges, and sometimes they would step in with their support to fill the void. During my time as a carer, I had access to and benefited from social interaction through clubs, social activities and friendships from closer relationships with other carers. Our relationship with our immediate neighbours also improved and strengthened.

I also found a new friend in Jenny through my Dementia journey and we formed a close friendship and now are writing our stories collaboratively.

I received enormous help with the packing up and gardening when I put my home up for sale from Maureen, who was also a carer herself and who had past experience running an aged care facility.

I have experienced that deep friendship with past carers who have already 'walked the walk', and are more sensitive in giving support.

Not only did I need Dementia support in the early days, but I craved it and these contacts resulted in lowering my stress levels. To understand Dementia I had to learn the following skills: I had to have a bucket load of patience, strong listening and planning skills, and most importantly the willingness to be flexible, as each of the Dementia stages evolved.

The Dementia expert advised carers to keep focus at all times on the abilities that remained and to stay in the present.

I considered myself extremely lucky to have had these learning opportunities from people who were not only experts in their fields, but they were there to help with Dementia strategies that worked, and we learnt ways to manage our care roles. The group of carers sometimes met socially and it helped to promote in a gentle way an acceptance of the disease.

An established routine in place helped somewhat to stay on top of things. But even the best routine brought its fair share of uncertainty. Jack had always followed a rigid routine and he still found comfort knowing what plans we had for the day. I would often find him checking the calendar daily. It is possible it reminded him of his working life. But Jack always seemed more at ease if his day ran to a routine and we had a good routine in place. Routine brought a little predictability, when the rest was all but gone.

Jack enjoyed the familiarity of his daily walks in our quiet neighbourhood. The walking paths were well designed and safe for his poor balance, and he enjoyed the peaceful scenery of the nature reserve. We would venture out each day on these short walks soon after breakfast, when he was at his most alert and relaxed. Sometimes we took another walk if I saw Jack needed a mood lift. It was amazing what a short walk can do for both the carer and the person living with Dementia!

As a carer, I soon found out there was no clock that even hinted at clock-off for the day!

Gardening had been Jack's passion and he continued with this activity when he lived at home, carrying on with tasks that he enjoyed. He watered and attended the annuals, and spent the best part of each day totally immersed in the activity of carrying pots from the front to back garden.

He was still able to take out the garbage, but the array of coloured bins confused him. Yet he could check out other bins lined up on the kerbside to get it right.

Jack still retained some awareness, bearing in mind he had good and bad days, although he was easily frustrated when his mind refused to prompt him and he would sigh frequently, 'my stupidity'!

They were also days when his concentration and memory would be so badly affected, and I saw such days as movie days at home, where he could nap, relax with a cup of tea, and feel normal and independent.

In the past Jack took much pride in his ability to hold a good conversation, even though English was his second language. In the period of his memory struggles, he found it extremely difficult to follow conversations in large groups, especially when conversation came at him from multiple directions. On the other hand, when his brain got systemically destroyed, he found it difficult to make sense of words and sounds in any language, even though he spoke several languages before he was impacted by the disease.

Jack's ability to use his autopilot had long disappeared, and made bedtime a daily challenge. I would sometimes have to turn his huge 195cm frame from a horizontal to a vertical position. I later discovered it was best to face him and gently push him on to the bed and jokingly say, 'Roll over.' This approach not only avoided a stressful moment but also avoided pointing out that he was wrong. I learnt this tip from Maureen, who was a matron at an aged care home.

Jack had also lost his ability to understand rules of a game when I would take his legs and turn him around, rather than explain he was lying in the wrong position. But he would react impatiently saying, 'Stop. I'm not a merry-go-round.'

I noticed his abilities disappeared in reverse order. Also I had no choice but to be consumed with his care 24/7, as Jack refused outside help. These increased care duties and his sole dependency on my time was exhausting, isolating and frightening.

Another bigger obstacle I faced as a carer was the perceived stigma attached to the disease. I often found myself hiding the diagnosis from friends because I was ashamed. This perception could have changed, if only I had better awareness measures in place at our early interventional stage of the disease. There is no traditional or social education happening in our society to understand Dementia positively, before the diagnosis is actually delivered.

Media reporting on Dementia matters is more negative and there are very few positive Dementia stories depicted as 'good news' stories. Nor is there enough Dementia conversation happening in our culture to understand what Dementia actually means. Rather than seeing Dementia as a mental illness or people living with Dementia as dangerous. Many other illnesses in our society invoke compassion and acceptance, as the disease is seen as a health issue.

Despite my ongoing struggles to care solely for Jack, I still found myself able to juggle caring, family and social commitments, when I started my Dementia education after the diagnosis was made.

Suddenly I had access to day care centres that provided much needed time out. Jack's attendance at the day care centres gave me the opportunity to attend Dementia courses in the community where I lived. These courses were especially run for carers to access services such as counselling and short respite stays. These short breaks gave me the boost to manage Jack's care at home for a bit longer.

The Dementia experts informed us that people who attend day care centres and respite care do adjust better when they are finally placed in a nursing home.

With the benefit of hindsight and with the positive Dementia community support services that I experienced, without hesitation I would now recommend that all Dementia carers should enrol in quality Dementia courses as soon as the Dementia diagnosis is delivered. I found that Dementia carer's support courses not only helped, but kept me informed, provided support services and numerous opportunities to meet other carers who had similar challenges in their daily lives. Importantly these different support groups sustained my care-giving experience.

As a past carer, I have subsequently learnt the road I travelled with Jack had many twist and turns. We were informed that carers save the governments huge sums of money and our care services were not budgeted in the health cost. So it is essential that carers stay vigilant and mindful of our own health care. We were reminded that there is a severe lack of respite care places in nursing homes, and it is extremely difficult to find emergency respite at short notice.

Additionally, my family was unable to step in as they had their own challenges and commitments!

The biggest stressor of Dementia caring was my daily communication with Jack. I had to learn new ways. I learnt that I could not talk from another room or while I walked with my back turned. At all times I had to face him to communicate simply, with few words. It had always been in Jack's personality to question the world around him, but to communicate with a faulty brain brought its own and different challenges. For Jack, as the disease progressed, he was no longer able to think straight, to stay focused or follow instructions.

Jack also had hearing problems, especially with background noise that interfered with his concentration, making normal conversation an on-going provocation.

Jack was often unable to follow and understand the reasons for my actions and he would accuse me of being deceitful or hiding the truth when he could not remember an appointment or visit, despite it being written in black and white on his daily calendar of events.

When I got thrown unexpectedly into the carer's job, I had little time to learn how to adjust to this mammoth job. Over time all of Jack's previous responsibilities became mine. For instance, I suddenly had to learn to manage our accounts as the posted reminders told me that Jack was now beyond managing our finances. The pile of late notices that appeared in the mail was proof enough. All charities that called our home were given endless amounts of cash. Whereas before Dementia he was a technology expert, and took care of all our media requirements, creating complicated databases, and collating music on different platforms and transferring all his music to his iTunes account, now he was unable to simply switch on the TV. He got confused with the numerous remote controls around him.

No one is born a 'carer'. I eased slowly into this care role, and I found it was a steep learning curve. Especially when the diagnosis was delivered, as there were countless medical appointments and services to arrange. I had to become Jack's advocate as his self-doubt increased and encourage his cooperation. I had to juggle both our lives and accept readily the sprinkling of failures and sins alike, as we both tried to live in the present.

I was thankful that Dementia shifted at a gradual pace. It helped me to cope and learn. Dementia stages moved with little warning from one stage to the next, and sometimes the stages would even overlap. The stages play out differently for each and every person living with Dementia. The gradual move of these early stages gave me the time to accept that the present situation would pass, and it was not my final destination.

Although both Jack and Fulton were diagnosed with Dementia with Lewy Bodies, the Dementia disease played out quite differently and uniquely for each of them. Dementia is not a one-size-fits-all model that can fit neatly in a box. It follows a unique progression for each individual.

Here are some tips that helped me enormously in my carer's role.

The mornings were particularly tough, with so much planning, as most appointments took place before lunch. I kept a diary that proved extremely useful and a 'do it list' that jolted my memory each day. Composing a list took time but the benefits I gained outweighed the time spent in designing it – and it helped Jack remain calm, knowing the plan for the next day.

I also kept a separate handwritten whiteboard with our weekly medical appointments, family and friend's visits.

I found telephones a time-waster and they went to message bank, that I screened later when time permitted.

I also planned one-pot meals that were easy to prepare and, on weekends, we treated ourselves to healthy takeaways.

All banking and grocery shopping was done online and delivered.

I readily accepted any offers of help and accepted Jeannette's offer in London to pay for Jack's respite services. It was a win–win for all. Jeannette felt involved in her father's care and I had a short break from caring. I found when I made reasonable and specific requests with the family it worked, as everyone knew what was required and they did not have to guess. Some of my friends volunteered to take Jack on short walks and outings and it gave me some time for myself.

I cannot emphasise how important it was that I learnt to streamline and prioritise the care duties each day. Despite good organisational strategies, I had little time to be a perfectionist. So I had to learn to lower my standards around the house and garden.

Another useful hint was to declutter. It helped with cleaning and also avoided accidents. I put a time limit on chores and this process helped to conserve both energy and precious time.

The most important rule I followed was flexibility. That helped to alleviate the carer's stress that had built up over the years.

It was only once the Dementia diagnosis was made that the GP connected and directed us to valuable community services that provided us with access to the local, state and national organisations. I found most of these community organisations were only a phone call away, and the highly trained staff were so willing to help novice carers to understand the Dementia disease. We touched on subjects such as:

- understanding why behaviour changes
- discovering stages of the dementia disease
- learning to care for yourself and your loved one
- recognising when it's time to seek additional care
- accepting grief, when you see how the disease changes the person you love.

I was lucky I had access to such good Dementia education, and I have listed below the resources that helped us to walk through the Dementia maze.

The Memory Clinic was attached to the local hospital, and a team of Dementia experts provided multidisciplinary services. It was the gerontologist initially who took Jack under her care, and treated us with utmost dignity and respect. She engaged with Jack to assess his Dementia stage and took notes on his personal history, his past profession, lifestyle, culture and preferences, including his likes, dislikes, hobbies or any other interests.

These notes then became a guide for the health professionals who worked in her team, to understand Jack's character and personality before the disease. Although this centre was not a medical or tertiary institution, the gerontologist worked closely with the research and development team. Jack only visited the Memory Clinic twice and the team specifically tailored Jack's treatment to meet his specific needs.

The best advice we received from the Memory Clinic was to participate in a variety of short courses that are run specifically in the community, to provide carers with valuable understanding and insight to Dementia care.

The Dementia education we received at these courses guided carers by transforming their grief or anger into more peaceful and hopeful feelings. We were informed that stress is caused when cognition deficits occur on a regular basis. And people who live with Dementia often wonder if they will ever get things right again, after the first go. This is unsettling for them.

The course presenters were mindful and gave equal support to the person with Dementia and their carers. We became a forum which shared openly with each other our Dementia experiences and the structured courses gave carers a voice to be heard, to be understood and carers were provided with workable clues to help manage Dementia care at home.

Many courses that the services ran would be of benefit to carers and we were invited to enrol in these courses if we were interested.

The first aid course was specifically designed to update carers' emergency skills.

The next was the legal course that made sure carers had their legal and financial matters under wraps. It was also brought to our notice the importance of the power of attorney and guardianships papers, which must be completed and signed long before the Dementia diagnosis is delivered, as legal documents lose their validity if made after the diagnosis. Help was provided to design an end-of-life care plan, and we were informed a well-designed care plan was like buying insurance before one dies.

The following were best-practice strategies that we were advised to apply when caring, and it helped many carers to provide better and holistic care at home.

The importance of regular visits to the family doctor was specifically stressed, as these visits managed the Dementia symptoms that occurred at different stages, and we were guided to access resources available in the community.

Time management, and food and nutrition advice was offered, and advice was given to ensure the pantry and freezer was always full and well stocked, for those busy and the unpredictable days.

An outline guide was delivered to carers so that we could recognise when it was time to seek additional help or to organise respite placement, so carers could get a break.

Issues relating to driving were discussed, like when it was time to stop before an accident happened.

Guidance and skills were provided to manage behavioural symptoms, and advice was provided to accept the new care role with positive understanding, and to allow time to adjust to caring, so that bitterness or grief would not to set in. Carers were informed of the importance to accept that the person you loved and had known for years was long gone, and accept that the partnership had now moved to one side.

We were advised to plan ahead with an employer, if still employed, so that employers had enough time to reschedule work changes at short notice. It helps carers not feel guilty when they have to take time off again.

I was also a carer to our grandchildren, two days a week, which I stopped when Jack's care demands became my priority.

Carers were encouraged to practise mindfulness techniques and we adopted these as part of our daily life, bringing great relief when caring posed difficulties. I used the slow breathing, while I repeated, 'There will be better days ahead', when caring became difficult.

Having access to a local Dementia support group in the neighbourhood helped me enormously. With their open-ended questions, we could recognise, support and celebrate each other's Dementia understanding, and the approaches we each chose to deliver care. I observed that carers demonstrated love for their partners. Their stories brought carers' strengths and resilience to the fore. The group's discussion and awareness made my own understanding of Dementia clearer. Group discussions gave the carers tools to cope, survive, heal the pain, and handle the emotional challenges that are a normal part of caring at home.

Even though we were unable to prevent an awful Dementia experience, we came out of the group discussion with a changed attitude, to carry on with our care duties when home. I found the advice on mindfulness skills beneficial: to be in the present, to focus and face one's partner when talking. It also helped to learn techniques of deep and slow breathing whilst holding one's own breath to a comfortable count when the situation became difficult. We were told it also helped to just leave the situation or take a short work outside, and to resume our presence only when calmness descended.

Jack's Dementia behaviours sometimes escalated to a rollercoaster ride, and it helped when I heard stories from other carers in a far worse care situation than my own. At times I felt like jumping off my seat and grabbing my own story from the circle and running! We were informed that it was okay to feel everything was rosy one minute and, in a few minutes, to have tears roll down uncontrollably for no apparent reason. We had a group coordinator, who did not have a personal Dementia experience, yet was competent to lead our carers' group to cultivate independent, objective and insightful perspectives.

Jack and I also enrolled in a specialised adult local day care centre that offered relief for carers, five days a week, for six hours a day. The centre observed school hours and holiday timetable. It was a secure and safe environment and the expenses incurred were absolutely worth the cost. Day care is hugely beneficial to carers, giving them time to enrol in Dementia awareness courses, and valuable time to reflect without interruptions, to unwind and for the body to adjust slowly.

The centre also gave carers an opportunity to connect with other people who had already been diagnosed with Dementia and meet other carers, at specially organised functions. I also noticed that each of the people attending the day care centre was at a different level in their Dementia stages.

The centre enabled me to have a short break from caring and Jack was able to retain his independence under supervised staff, who helped him to engage in activities that still remained intact and which stimulated his brain, to do puzzles and to read the paper. But Jack was unable to engage socially with the staff or the other attendees.

Another advantage of attending such centres, is that it was not just me doing all the reminding. I had support from the staff who also enforced the same values, of good hygiene, water drinking, and reminded Jack to close the doors. I especially welcomed the hot lunches that were served each day. That meant I could plan a simple and light evening meal five days a week and not feel guilty. Another welcome relief was a weekend respite care that Jack received once a month. He was dropped off on Friday morning and collected after lunch on Sunday.

I just count myself lucky that I found Jenny and received community support and information from another carer who was on the same Dementia experience as myself. I rang her each evening and Jenny would relate her actual experiences by storytelling when she was still caring for Fulton at home. I am pleased I did not have to depend solely on Dementia books for my awareness, or get my understanding by reading academic research papers.

Jenny lived in Canberra whilst I resided in Sydney. Jenny had just placed Fulton in a nursing home, whereas I had just received the Dementia diagnosis, when we first made our contact.

We stayed in contact using social media each day to communicate, using technologies like the telephone, text messaging, emails, internet searches and reading blogs. The nights were the hardest for us both, as that was when our fear and isolation descended, with the house quiet and our husbands in bed. I would discuss my group meeting and the stories I heard, or sometimes talk of Jack's progress or decline.

Jenny wished she had had the same access, when she first took on the carer's role for Fulton. Jenny too started her care role in the dark, and by the time Fulton received his diagnosis, he had already reached the 'high-care' stage and Jenny was unable to leave Fulton to attend any meetings.

In our email exchange and diaries that we each kept, we wrote our daily thoughts, doubts and experiences, identified workable and unworkable decisions, and freely discussed points that we may have overlooked. We discussed how difficult it was to work in the dark in the early days.

But it was easier for me, as Jenny willingly took me under her wing and shared the positive and negative lessons she had learnt from her Dementia understanding as a carer. This meant that I would not have to experience the pain she endured without the level of professional or group support available to me in Sydney. I sometimes wonder if carers living in regional centres have the same level of support and access that we in the city are privileged to have.

Jenny delivered an excellent human-to-human connection and helped me to ease into a carer's role from the start to the end of living with Dementia. Our meeting only happened after Jack died. This connection was critical to both our mind frame, even though we both walked and experienced Dementia differently, as we each had different needs as the disease unfolded.

Jenny's lived Dementia experiences became an excellent opportunity to talk plainly to another carer, with total honesty and few inhibitions on my part, and this made my caring at home less painful. Jenny gave me the luxurious gift of Dementia empowerment, by healing the emotional scars I carried without medication or professional counselling. Jenny's positive approach helped enormously and became the reason to share our stories and to inspire other carers to seek support from members in the community who have already experienced the pain and as a result have valuable hindsight.

I was introduced to Jenny by a mutual friend, who also lived in Canberra, and had the insight not to give advice on a subject she had little knowledge. She saw Jenny as the ideal person to help me move forward and to ease my stress, largely due to my ignorance of the disease when the diagnosis was delivered.

Before Jenny came on the scene, I was extremely angry and unable to express my acute grief. After much discussion on each other's beliefs and values, I learnt anger was a natural way to exhibit grief and she motivated me to push through the tough circumstances and I had to see the light, to be ready and to accept the reality of Dementia.

Jenny further informed me that patience and a positive attitude was what helped her get through the difficult days, as she too was fearful and harboured negative thoughts with no one to talk to and to show understanding. She pointed out that children actually do not want to hear the sad tales, nor do parents want to burden or shift the memory of their father which their children cherished. She said, 'Dementia is a long wait', and in the meantime she had learnt to tame her anger and frustration.

Acceptance was the key to make life liveable for both Jack and myself. But acceptance of a Dementia diagnosis was difficult to accept when Jack did not look ill. Sometimes I put his character changes down to becoming a 'grumpy' old man. But seeing his memory loss that I alone was privy to each day was enough proof that it was not possible for Jack to give up the independence that he cherished!

The social and medical support I experienced from Jenny and the medical health professionals was the kickstart to my healing process. To accept the illness. There was no point in disagreeing with the person living with Dementia, as it only brought bitterness.

When certain parts of the brain got damaged with Dementia advancing, behavioural challenges manifested. Stages of Dementia were not linear and Jack moved from an easy to a difficult stage in minutes. I used his behaviours as a marker to prepare emotionally for Jack's next decline by seeing the GP on our return from Europe to make arrangements for care placement in a nursing home.

Jack's Dementia with Lewy Bodies is an umbrella term to describe a group of symptoms that affected various parts of Jack's brain, and which often made him feel less useful or in control. Dementia is a complex disease and acutely affected his brain and he sometimes experienced loss of his motor skills. This would vastly alter his personality and interfered with the way he led his day-to-day life.

Jack was diagnosed with mixed Dementia, a condition that represented more than one type of Dementia and with changes occurring simultaneously in his brain. Dementia with Lewy Bodies generally explained his behavioural issues, but despite knowing the reason, it was still not easy to accept readily when disturbing episodes occurred without warning.

The best marker of Dementia in Jack's case was his slow decline from one celebration event to the next, and the steady loss of his abilities was easily noticed. To Jeannette who lived in London and who visited every six months, Jack's decline was more obvious.

While memory loss played a major part in the damage to Jack's brain, he also had acute loss with three out of the five senses, which played a huge part in the limitations on him enjoying life as he knew it. The loss of hearing also made conversation difficult especially when in a group and when conversation came at him from all directions. Finally he lost his sense of smell. He failed to smell his food burning on the stove – and he doused the pan with petrol, starting a small fire in the kitchen. He masked these signs by painting the whole kitchen! I then realised Jack could no longer be left at home unsupervised.

The underlying cause for his delirium and hallucinatory behaviours was often the result of a urinary tract infection (UTI) which sometimes could be the start of psychotic delusions. With Jack's Dementia advancing he would experience occasional hallucinations. They appeared to be real in his mind. These delusions were largely perceptions not based on any reality, often appearing rapidly. They would leave Jack confused and the behaviours would affect his thinking. In some people the hallucinations may be temporary, or persist over a long term, largely depending upon the exact type of hallucinations and their causes.

Jack had such an episode when he was on the operating table and under anaesthetic. He saw people coming to attack him. Sometimes he would hear sounds, or feel a sensation as if ants were crawling on his body, or he would smell odours that were not there. Most of his hallucinations would take place at night, and he would lash out and jump out of bed.

A UTI would also raise his body temperature, and sometimes it had an effect on his balance as well, which led to several falls. Initially I would call an ambulance as I was unable to lift Jack off the floor. But then I learnt a technique from Maria to use a steady chair, which Jack held, as he supported himself off the floor.

This is a story of a delusional attack and a common feature of a severely damaged brain that took years to manifest and the episodes played rapidly and disappeared as suddenly as the delusion appeared. In 2013 Jeannette invited us to have a European summer in Tuscany with her young family, as she did not want to take the long trip to Sydney with them. Jack's brother Alphons and his wife Mieke would also join us on this holiday. The earlier plan in place was Jack's wish that I should travel on my own to Italy for two weeks. He felt it was beyond him to embark on such a long holiday to Europe, that involved hours of travel and he was happy to stay home under the supervision of a paid carer.

In the past, Jack's decisions came from a predictable and rational place, and he always made sure he had controls in place so he could call the shots. However, I failed to realise that the new person I now lived with had dysfunctional tendencies, along with increasingly unpredictable behaviours.

Old beliefs and habits die hard! With Jack's conversation normal his wish made total sense and I failed to notice the uncertainty of the Dementia disease.

With so much sadness in a Dementia household, I grabbed at any normalcy. To me this conversation was normal, rational and our marriage vows resonate 'for better or worse'.

A month before I left for Europe, I organised for the paid carer to come and stay with Jack, whilst I went away on a long weekend for a short break. The trial care plan was successful.

But two weeks before my trip, Jack decided to have a change of mind and announced that he would join me on the holiday to Europe. He pointed out, 'I am unwilling to spend two weeks dining with a stranger at my table, and have decided to join you.' Of course I was delighted he was making this huge effort, without any pressure from any members of the family. Jack could be described as a determined person, a warm, loving and devoted husband, father and Opa, who was keen to spend time with his family, possibly knowing it would be his last visit to Europe.

The GP and gerontologist both confirmed it was safe for Jack to travel, as this holiday was largely with familiar family members and our stay would be largely in private homes, with limited use of public transport. Besides one long flight to Europe and two short flights to Holland and back to Italy.

During this period Jack was still doing well in a social situation, and could have normal and nonspecific conversation. Jack was still totally engaged with his immediate family and surrounding neighbours, and sometimes took his morning walks on his own without missing a beat. He engaged enthusiastically with our grandchildren when we babysat in our home. If he struggled to find a word momentarily, a simple prompt would enable him to weave back into the conversation. He still talked with orientation, used family names correctly, discussed the present, still able to discuss current events, still able to read time correctly, still managed to catch the right train on his own to the city and back, still able to follow a train timetable, still coped with crowds on his own, and still came home safely without an incidents. That was because Dementia typically destroys memories in reverse order, the long-term social skills of his past along with the learnt knowledge of past still intact.

We travelled business class and Jack coped well with the long travel. He slept for most of the long trip. However, for a person living with Dementia, I knew his behaviour could change quickly and suddenly. He could act quite differently from a few hours or even days before. The long and hazardous travel experience from Sydney to Milan tested my emotional resilience. The trip became turbulent and stormy on landing at Milan airport and, within minutes of our arrival, I was faced with challenging behaviours. My immediate reaction was to automatically run away and save myself from the embarrassing incident that followed.

Suddenly Jack became extremely suspicious and refused to budge any further, after we completed our immigration check. I was able to distract his attention and move him to the information desk. He did not shout, swear or lash out at me or the staff. Jack was a respectful and a reasonable gentleman always. His personality changed because he was totally exhausted after his long flight to the other end of the world and confused in the strange environment where he found himself.

When we reached the information desk, Jack declared to the receptionist that he was abducted, and I was an imposter, and he had been brought to Europe against his will. I handed a card to the receptionist that read, 'My husband has Dementia'.

She called the police who were thoughtful, caring and respectful, and had Jack sitting in a wheelchair and, within minutes, he seemed totally relaxed. It could be possible his legs were stiff and wobbly after sitting for hours on the long trip, and he was unable to verbalise that he could not walk the endless airport corridors to get to the immigration queue.

This is what a delusional behaviour looks like. It was Jack's way of saying, 'I am tired and now want to go home.'

Most hurtful were his delusional episodes when he saw me as an imposter.

Dementia awareness helped me get out of a very sticky situation. It was Dementia understanding that highlighted that a carer has always to remain centred, regardless of what the circumstances or situation. The job of a carer was always to be emotionally present, to be an advocate and take full responsibility for the situation presented.

The episode only lasted a few minutes and disappeared as quickly as it happened.

It is a good example of Dementia at play – one minute relaxed and the next, a totally unpredictable person that often brought tears of frustration. I did not distract Jack's attention to another situation or another activity, nor did I take offence, argue or try to convince him otherwise. I stayed calm throughout the whole act, and made sure I quietly and slowly took deep breaths through the nose, and exhaled through the mouth while I watched the delusional behaviour play its course. I think I was relaxed as the people around the airport went about their own business. Neither Jack nor I made a scene. Events like these leave carers totally done and this time it was a double whammy, a result of extreme tiredness and the long air trip to Europe.

At last Jack was sitting totally relaxed. It seemed like the police had sedated him, rather than simply providing him with a wheelchair to rest. The two police kindly accompanied us to the taxi stand and we drove away to our hotel. Jack occupied the front seat of the taxi and once seated, requested the taxi driver, 'Please drive us to Sydney and I will pay you $100.'

I again handed the Dementia card to the taxi driver. He read the text written in Italian – I was totally prepared, along with the hotel details. The taxi driver drove away without commenting.

Here was an ample proof that although Jack looked and behaved well for most of the trip, only a little trigger to his damaged brain brought about a delusional attack. Delusional behaviours are not intentionally designed to annoy. When the challenging behaviour took place at Milan airport, I felt so 'alone' and the marriage vows resonated, 'Until death do us part ...' again.

Again, the Dementia community programs that I attended had given me the insight to understand Dementia. They were specifically designed for carers to understand behaviours in a practical ways and to defuse situations with compassion, by means of using a gentle approach, rather than sedation or physical restraints. A gentle and caring approach was what achieved the peaceful end.

When we reached our hotel, Jack rested and the agitated episode left no sign when he woke. We left our hotel room in the direction of the tourist office so we could explore the wonderful and magnificent surrounds of Lake Como where our hotel was situated. To reach the tourism information office, we had to climb a few comfortable stairs, but halfway into our climb Jack suddenly fell backwards. Luckily a tourist who was a doctor was also in the queue, went on his knees to check Jack over and advised me to leave him on the ground until he was ready to get up on his own. On leaving, the doctor advised that I should make an appointment for a local doctor to visit our hotel room and check him over before he went to bed.

The GP who checked Jack over was unimpressed, and accused the Australian medical staff and myself for being totally irresponsible. I was particularly selfish to take a person already living with Dementia to embark on such a long trip to the other end of the world.

It surprised me even further to learn from the visiting GP that Jack's behavioural reaction was a chemical imbalance in his brain. The doctor explained, 'The low air pressure that is associated when flying thins the blood, which can sometimes strengthen the effects and bring about delusional behaviour.'

He went on to say, 'During a long flight, the barometric pressure in the cabin is always lower than it is in most places on earth, and the decreased pressurised environment diminishes the body's ability to absorb oxygen.'

The doctor also brought to my attention that a person with Dementia's body is slower to adjust to the outside air and the challenging behaviours go into action immediately and disappear as suddenly as they appear. And this information was also correct.

The episode only lasted for 15 minutes and the doctor prescribed medication and we spent two days in Lake Como taking in the sights at a leisurely pace.

The doctor also checked if Jack was properly hydrated when he travelled on this long flight to Europe. He said it was important as aircrafts release dry air, and could cause dehydration. I was advised that I should continue with the water drinking for a few more days. And if alcohol was consumed, it was advised, a glass of water should be consumed for every glass wine that was drunk.

Another episode unfolded in Milan when I thoughtlessly asked Jack to sit out in the fresh air and wait while I made a quick dash to the bank to get local currency. I was only away for less than five minutes, and when I came out Jack had already disappeared. On checking the street, I noticed a tall gentleman taking in the beautiful sights of Lake Como and I quickly hurried to catch up as he was casually walking amongst the crowds of tourists.

Then we drove from Lake Como to Florence in a hired car with a driver, which was arranged by Jeannette so I could keep an eye on Jack. The driver drove around the lake whilst we took in the scenic surrounds. We enjoyed the lake's views with its renowned crystal clear water and the surrounding alpine mountains that were dotted by medieval and baroque buildings all the way to Florence. Our trip to Florence went smoothly and Jeannette then took on the caring role for her father and I had the responsibility to care for our young grandchildren.

Dementia does not allow the luxury to think or plan ahead. After years of caring, I learnt to take each day at a time and sometimes days could get very creative, and very varied when on the run. What worked one day does not still work the next day. Dementia throws out predictability and even a well organised routine goes out the window.

Another hint is to always ensure pain is managed properly, as this avoids a vicious cycle of a bad day turning into a string of bad days.

On arriving at the Tuscan villa, Jack had another delusional attack. On seeing the villa, he refused to get out of the car saying to Jeannette, 'I do not have this sort of money.' He was under the impression Jeannette had bought the villa and expected him to pay.

Somehow, our daughter managed to get him out of the car, without arguing or displaying frustration or anger. She matter-of-fact stated, 'Dad, you have lived in London long enough to know, there is no guarantee to experience a summer, that is why we have come to Italy to get some sun. Besides, I know you specifically moved to Australia for the sun. So let us get out and together experience a Tuscan summer, of food and wine.' Our daughter defused a tense situation by her casual and accepting approach. In Europe, his visual hallucinations were different, it was not people or animals this time, it was villas!

The sub-set of Dementia with Lewy Bodies was now affecting Jack's motor ability to get out of the car and walk up to the front door. Jack's days of anxious behaviour brought on the Parkinson's symptoms, manifesting as stiffness and his legs became rigid, slow and hesitant. He was unable to walk the slight incline to the front door. Our daughter and son-in-law then assisted and guided him up the driveway, by each of them holding him under the arm.

During the day Jack's behaviour was normal. The family kept the communication channels open by sharing their daily experiences and this made Jack feel he was heard and understood. For example, our daughter adopted a conscientious and mindful way to be his carer, and accepted the new care role without debate. She eased into the new caregiving role by ensuring I stayed nearby. I cannot recommend this independent and objective approach strongly enough. It was supportive – and a learning tool that worked.

Our week's stay in Tuscany was positive. We all stayed calm and relaxed and Jack even interacted and played football with our young grandchildren. There was no sign of impaired cognition, lack of initiative or interest, or diminished alertness. His past traveller's experience became obvious. Jack fully enjoyed the scenic drives, our daily morning walks with the extended family, followed with coffee on the terrace, whilst we watched the activities of the ancient market place. While at the villa, Jack assisted with the meal preparation and conversed normally with our daughter. But at night he still wanted our daughter to be around while he organised his bedtime routine.

Our daughter focused on what was not lost. At all times she helped her father to stay calm and distracted him by talking about the simple plans she had arranged for the next day. Jack felt reassured and safe. She held his hands when he showed traces of anxiety, rather than use words.

After a week's stay in Italy we made a short plane trip to visit his family in Holland and our intention was to return to Tuscany with Jack's brother Alphons and his wife Mieke for another two weeks before we flew home to Sydney.

The short flight from Italy to Holland was uneventful. The pressurised air on the plane did not take a toll on Jack's brain on this short trip. Jack appeared extremely happy and immediately settled seeing his brother Alphons. I noticed his memory was connected to his past childhood memories long formed when he was young.

He again enjoyed the Dutch way of life and remarked as we pulled out of the car park, 'Look around, how everything is clean, orderly, and the streets are clearly sign-posted.' This consciousness was learnt in the past and developed through his childhood, and it was interesting that it still remained intact. Or maybe a clear mind was easier to maintain in a Dutch orderly landscape!

Once with his siblings, the family took total charge and I had time off to be a tourist with my sister-in-law Mieke. Despite welcoming the free time, there was loneliness. Although we still had each other, companionship as we had known it was long over and I slowly learnt to surrender, rather than resist.

Jack in the meantime continued to be extremely conscientious and happy in his Dutch surrounds. He thoroughly enjoyed the company of his siblings, and he was happy to re-live the memories he shared with them as a child. He visited his childhood haunts, school, the neighbourhood where he grew up, relished the Dutch cuisine and generally reminisced about his happy childhood memories.

His siblings did notice his short-term memory loss – but Jack was still able to hide or mask his symptoms and engage in show time. There were no mood swings, paranoia or any signs of depression or anxiety whilst on his short visit to Holland. I also arranged another GP visit in Holland to make sure Jack was well enough to continue a further two weeks in Europe and the Dutch doctor gave him a clear bill of health.

On our return to Tuscany, with Alphons and Mieke in tow, Dementia with Lewy Bodies made another visit and ruled our life again. On days like this, most carers would like to either hide or simply run away. Jack informed our daughter that, having spent a memorable week with her and her family and now that he had seen his family in Holland, it was time he departed for home in Sydney. We all kept calm. Knowing there was no point in arguing, disagreeing or creating another drama.

Jack's Dementia had already robbed him of his presence as a warm and caring family member and this irrational behaviour made the fate of those he loved, uniquely heart wrenching.

Jack and I went upstairs to pack our suitcases. I did not interfere with his packing, even when I noticed he struggled. I let him be and thought it best to complete the packing when he left the room.

Our daughter had to change our departure dates for a small administration fee, otherwise we had no problem changing the date on our return ticket. The trip to Milan airport took two hours by car from our Tuscan villa, and our daughter and Alphons drove us to Milan Airport.

My reaction at having to go home early brought both sadness and anger, at life and everyone who gave us advice that it was okay to travel to the other side of the world. Jack had already been diagnosed with Dementia for two years. I did not see the point in showing how disappointed and shattered I was. I was especially hurt to leave the grandchildren who were just beginning to get relaxed in my company. Nevertheless

I took solace while I showered to silently scream – and it helped!

The family, including the young children, had to take a back seat while Jack became the focus of this trip. At least I had some good memories to cherish, the happy times spent with our daughter and her family in Tuscany, and the love and care Jack received from his family in Holland. I was also grateful that Jack had an opportunity to experience a final hometown visit and the care and kindness he was surrounded by on this visit with his family.

At the airport we sat in silence while we watched the incoming and departing flights, sipping our coffee in the lounge. I took his hand and reassured him of my presence in silence. At the same time I prayed silently not to experience another delusional episode at Sydney airport. But luckily our long trip home was uneventful.

***

Jenny and Blanche's tips:
Caring at home

- Get informed and educate yourself in understanding Dementia as it moves through several stages over many years and sometimes the stages overlap.
- Join Dementia courses run by Dementia Australia as you get to learn from experts in the field.
- Find day care and neighbourhood centres in the community, to learn from other carers. They are also a useful place to get to know about what resources are available for all Dementia sufferers and their carers.
- Establish a daily routine.
- Use a whiteboard to display the daily schedule.

- Keep a notebook to record all relevant information about the person for whom you are caring, eg doctors' contact details, nursing home observations, etc.
- Prepare the next day's clothing needs and hang on the bedroom door.
- Implement 'distraction methods' to defuse tantrums.
- Arrange regular respite care.
- Allow family and friends to help on regular basis.
- Create an 'information card' to be carried by the person for whom you are caring. This should have contact details, including address of next of kin, and identify the carrier as a person with Dementia.
- Buy a mobile GPS watch for seniors, to be worn at all times.
- Remind the person with Dementia of the need to have regular toilet breaks.
- Try to arrange regular rest breaks for yourself, away from the person for whom you are caring.

Chapter 3

Nursing home choice

JENNY AND FULTON'S STORY

Dear Blanche
I never thought having to choose a nursing home in which to place Fulton permanently would ever be one of my life experiences. Dementia, I now learnt, doesn't allow choices, and the guilt is mine to bear ...

***

Hopefully, you will learn from Blanche and me a few things which may assist you in looking for and making your final choice of an appropriate nursing home for the person for whom you are caring.

Blanche and Jack had a totally different experience with nursing home choice from that which Fulton and I experienced. Blanche was fortunate in that her search did not involve as many 'detours' as mine, and it proved to be successful from the start. Blanche had a much better outcome due to a totally serendipitous meeting. By chance and good luck she met a doctor's wife at an Alzheimer's conference who told her how pleased she had been with the nursing home where her husband had recently spent two years, before passing away from Dementia.

Blanche followed up on this recommendation and eventually placed Jack there. However, prior to this meeting she had done a lot of preliminary searching herself first, so she was well-informed on Jack's needs and her own. On investigating this recommendation Blanche found the nursing home fulfilled all their requirements.

Jack passed away after living there for two years. Blanche was impressed with the level of care he received at all times.

Her only issue involved him escaping and going missing in the city for a few hours! This highlights a real need to ensure the security of your chosen nursing home is water-tight.

Fulton did not manage to ever escape from his various short-term respite care facilities, nor from his full-time nursing home, but this was not from want of trying!

However I did make a point of reviewing the security protocols for high-care patients before Fulton stayed in any of them. As his primary carer I was conscious that it was my duty to ensure Fulton would be completely safe when living away from our home.

I must say he tried to escape from each place on numerous occasions by being quite devious. He would hang around the exit door just waiting for a chance to run, but he was never successful.

It seems this desire to escape or run away is a common characteristic of most people with Dementia. The first time it happens can be terrifying to the carer and all the family. Sadly, some such escapades can have the worst outcome thinkable, as no doubt you are already aware.

Fulton's nursing home journey was certainly less straight-forward than Jack's had been. We experienced a couple of difficult detours along the way. I found every step in choosing a nursing home challenging, but tried to bring about the best outcome for Fulton. I wanted him to live the last stage of his life in a safe and secure, caring environment.

I certainly did not foresee the problems we encountered, which proved to be the most challenging and traumatic parts of our Dementia journey.

Assessing which nursing homes are suitable for your needs, as a primary carer, and which ones suit the Dementia needs of the person you are caring for, is an extremely important part of the Dementia journey.

It may seem strange to even think of your needs, but it is important to take into consideration things like your travel time from your family home to the nursing home, as you may be fulfilling this role for some time. You will visit regularly so you probably will not want to travel for hours to get there. You also need to check out what areas are set aside for visitors.

Some nursing homes only have a chair in a bedroom where you can sit beside the person you are visiting, for example. This would make it challenging if a few family members wish to visit at the same time.

Additionally, I would recommend discussing with your 'potential' nursing home staff, what their 'pandemic' protocols are (no surprises!).

At Fulton's nursing home, there were several private areas where we could spend time together. I especially enjoyed sitting with Fulton in the tranquil garden areas. When you are surrounded by a number of high-care patients, it is so important to have a private and quiet area where you can escape the daily noise, and sometimes chaos of a high-care unit.

Blanche visited Jack daily for years and I visited Fulton regularly over five months. Both of us did not have far to travel for our visits which proved to be a godsend. These visits can be physically and emotionally draining, so it is good to be able to return home quickly and easily each day.

Perhaps you may need to sell the family home to fund a nursing home placement for your husband. Then you will need to think of where you want to reside in the future. You do not need to be facing long travel distances to visit a husband or family member, so this is why you need to be practical about choosing the nursing home which suits you.

Once you have found a couple of location options you should list them in order of preference. Sometimes the need for a nursing home placement may occur unexpectedly, so it is imperative you have a few on your list from which to choose. Another reason it is essential to list more than one suitable nursing home is your preferred choice may not have a vacancy available when the need arises. Many nursing homes have lengthy waiting lists so put your name down as soon as possible on a couple of lists, as it is better to have multiple options to choose from.

I had mistakenly believed I could care for Fulton at home until he died. When I thought this, I had no idea of what was involved in being a full-time Dementia carer over an extended period of time! In the early stages of Dementia, I did not understand just how challenging the disease would become. I thought I could manage caring for Fulton until the end of his life, possibly by employing nursing staff to help me.

This is the reason I did not look for a nursing home immediately after the Dementia diagnosis. This was a big mistake which I encouraged Blanche not to repeat.

I quickly discovered that our home was not equipped to provide for the physical needs of a person in the final stages of

Dementia. Nor was I strong enough to cope with the physical demands of lifting Fulton several times a day in and out of bed and helping him to stand after one of his frequent falls.

It was not an easy decision and one which I procrastinated over for as long as I could. At times I was consumed by guilt at the idea of sending Fulton away to be cared for by strangers. However as every day passed, I realised I was becoming less able to deal with the confronting and challenging behaviours which are characteristic of high care Dementia: aggression, hallucinations, insomnia and anti-social antics.

Watching the person you love disintegrate, slowly at first, before your eyes, takes a special type of resilience. A daughter or son caring for a parent who is not living with them would most likely have to put their parent into full-time care a lot earlier than I did with Fulton. Had Fulton been living at home alone, I have no doubt he would have wandered off or electrocuted himself accidentally, or maybe burnt the house down.

High-care Dementia patients need 24-hour supervision for their own safety – and that of their personal carers. So prepare for moving your family member as soon as possible after diagnosis.

Waiting lists can be long and organising the financial administrative arrangements may take months. I just could not believe how complicated the forms were to complete. It took me hours and although I have several university degrees, I had never had to do anything as complicated as that before. In comparison a passport application is a breeze. So I suggest allowing a significant amount of time for this particular task as it is one that you cannot hurry.

I recommend you start to do some research as soon as possible after diagnosis, even before you think a nursing home admission may be ever needed.

Do consider consulting with your local Alzheimer's or Dementia association for whatever services they have to offer to help you in this regard. Also it may be useful to consult a professional nursing home consultant who, at a cost, can advise you on the many aspects of this journey. There are a lot of administrative tasks involved in this process so having a qualified consultant to assist you may be well worth the initial cost involved. However, in the end, you and your family will have to make the final choice.

Blanche and I decided not include specific details concerning the financial cost of paying for full-time nursing home care in our story. In Australia there is great variability in the cost of nursing home care from state to state.

Also, all families have different financial situations. What may be a terrible drain for one family, may not even make a dint in another family's financial resources.
In addition, cultural and social practices vary considerably between different families. In some families, all the children may contribute to the cost of a parents nursing home fees. Whilst in another family the spouse pays for everything.

Although we had always been financially comfortable and saved for our future life together, Fulton and I had not factored in the significant cost of long-term nursing home residence or in-home costs of hiring carers when we had done our long-term retirement (pre-Dementia) financial planning. Mainly because we had not foreseen Dementia care being a part of our future.

This is one of the unspoken major stresses that the spouse and family of a Dementia patient have to cope with. Losing a spouse to a terminal illness is hard enough, but possibly having to sell and leave the family home with all its related memories may also be traumatic. Especially when it occurs under such difficult circumstances.

The trauma of losing a spouse or family member is still the hardest part of this situation, whether financial difficulties have to be overcome or not.

Moving your spouse into a nursing home is just another aspect of this illness which has been rightly defined as 'the long goodbye'. It must be heartbreaking for those who lose their husband's company due to the necessity of a nursing home placement, but also have to leave the home they have lived in together for many years.

Dementia can be quite a cruel journey.

The guilt which most spouse carers may feel in finally deciding they are no longer able to care for their family member – in my case my husband – may seem unbearable. I felt I was betraying Fulton, as we had both always said living permanently in a nursing home was not really living at all. Acknowledging that I was no longer capable of looking after Fulton's needs was hard for me to accept.

As his Dementia progressed, even having a couple of hours paid carer help per day was not enough to guarantee Fulton's personal care and safety, or my own, over a 24-hour period. His night-time wanderings both inside and outside the home ensured I had little rest. Nor was it safe to have our front-door open and unlocked regularly, when he took off on one of his unannounced middle-of-the-night escape expeditions.

We must have looked a funny sight wandering around our local suburb in night attire. He behaved like a naughty puppy that had jumped a fence and escaped. As soon as I got close to catching him, pleading with him to come home, he would take off in another direction. Fortunately, fatigue would take over eventually and the offer of a coffee sometimes enticed him home – especially if it was a cold night!

One way I alleviated my guilt at placing Fulton in a nursing home was to convince myself I could search for and find the best possible nursing home available for him. I had realised it needed to be nearby, but I also knew it had to have the capability of providing for his Dementia needs, in an appropriate compassionate and caring way.

Although I told the children I was doing a search for the perfect nursing home for their father, I did not ask them to participate directly in the search, or to come to the preliminary interviews. I did tell them what I was doing but I felt they had their own lives to live and did not want to burden them with any more problems or sadness. They often helped me by sitting at home with their father, so I was free to go alone on my searches. However, I welcomed any input they wanted to make to this project.

I tried to be totally objective and calm about this sad task. But as Fulton deteriorated before my eyes, there was hardly a day I did not lie in bed at night weeping silent tears at our situation. My sadness and guilt were for him and what might have been. There was to be no happy twilight years for us, only daily anguish, at the struggle Dementia causes in just living day to day.

I was angry and guilty at the same time. Why Fulton? Why us? It was especially hard to listen to friends of our age planning their overseas jaunts and future shared plans. Our only outings over the past few years had been to visit family and doctors, or a walk to the local shops. We had no joint future. Our planned retirement years had turned to dust. The lines from Shakespeare were constantly in my mind, 'I wasted time and now doth time waste me.'

But being resilient and positive at that time, I tried not share my true feelings with anyone, except later with Blanche, particularly as my children were having to cope with the gradual loss of their father. I know they did not need to see me fall apart. I tried to direct all their care and support to their father. Although they frequently asked me if I was okay, I kept telling them I was fine, and to a certain extent I was.

The support our children gave us both, was amazing. They really kept me going by popping in to see me regularly and taking us out at least once a week. The grandchildren's chatter and stories about school and friends lifted my spirits considerably.

I think the hardest part of the nursing home journey is, having exhausted all other possibilities, making the final decision you can no longer care for your husband, wife, sister or brother. This decision is so hard.

I had decided I would look after Fulton for as long as I was physically and emotionally able. I am a resilient person and had decided immediately after the diagnosis that I would do this because it was the right thing to do. After all, I had promised to be by his side 'for richer, for poorer, in sickness and in health, till death us do part'. However, I am not Mother Teresa, and when I found he became too challenging to live with and was unable to carry out the most basic tasks relating to hygiene, like showering and toileting, I realised it was time to start considering the alternatives to 'at home' care.

My children became worried about my health, as the caring role was taking its toll. There is no respite for the carer, from the 24-hour a day care of a Dementia-impacted person. I started to use agency carers to come into our home twice daily to help me.

Fulton hated strangers being in the home and sometimes was rude to them. I found them to be wonderful caring people who were as kind and considerate to me, as they were to Fulton. But his initial slow decline now accelerated and the carers indicated Fulton would need full-time care soon. This was not just due to his sometimes volatile behaviour, but also that he needed equipment to lift him in and out of bed which I did not have in our home.

They suggested I place Fulton into a respite care facility, to see how he coped and to give myself a short break. I did this and the time alone made me realise that I now had to focus on finding a nursing home for Fulton.

I put as much effort into choosing a safe, comfortable nursing home for Fulton to live in, as I had done years before when I had undertaken research in choosing a school for my children. Similarly, Alycia and Olli recently spent many months looking for a suitable place for their son Otto for childcare. This reminded me of the process I needed to undertake to find a suitable caring, safe environment for Fulton. Like babies in a childcare institution, high-care Dementia patients are particularly vulnerable, as they may lack the ability to report neglect, cruelty or lack of care. Many high-care patients become non-verbal as the Dementia progresses to the final stages.

As the primary carer, our caring role does not terminate when your husband, wife, partner or family member enters a nursing home. You still have duty of care. You will find yourself watching out for their wellbeing every day when you visit. I do believe you have to be extra vigilant and on alert for bad practice.

Sadly, the Royal Commission into Aged Care in Australia has revealed many cases where little compassion or care has been shown to Dementia patients. Some of the hearings and submissions made to the Royal Commission highlighted Dementia patient abuse and neglect. Nursing homes which may appear on the surface to look attractive caring institutions with qualified empathetic staff have sometimes been the worst offenders against their most vulnerable residents.

Just remember everything may not be as it seems to be! A beautifully designed and attractively decorated nursing home with smiling efficient staff does not necessarily translate into being the best place for the person for whom you are providing care.

Sadly, I discovered this myself when Fulton had to leave the very first nursing home I had chosen after just one night, despite all my careful research. So be extra vigilant when you are visiting the nursing homes prior to making your final choice. I spent a great deal of time doing these preliminary visits so I could feel confident that when I made my final choice, I would know it was the best residence for Fulton's end-of-life care.

I really had done all I could do to ensure he would be safe and well cared for by trained professionals. I needed to go to bed each night knowing I had done my best to choose a home where Fulton would be safe, well cared for and comfortable.

So my reasons for choosing a suitable nursing home had been flawed.

What went wrong? I thought I had done the most thorough research possible.

Unfortunately, when I first attended the nursing homes, I really did not know enough about Dementia and how it progressed to ask the right questions. I certainly would not have predicted the escalation of Fulton's Dementia-related behaviours. Initially I thought Fulton would just decline slowly. Also, when we both attended interviews, Fulton's appearance belied the fact that he was in every possible way a high-care patient. His behaviour was impeccable when I was by his side.

At the time we were going for medical appointments, he was living at home and was mainly calm and relaxed. He appeared to be a high-functioning older person. He was most presentable, a handsome man, with piercing blue eyes and a full head of wavy grey hair. I ensured he was well-groomed and dressed immaculately – no baggy track suits or sneakers for him. So he was still able to make a good first impression.

Although he could no longer read or write, he was polite and certainly not violent or aggressive, nor had he ever been during the early stages of his illness. His language skills had diminished, but he could still communicate in a very basic way.

He could mask his true feelings for about 20 minutes before having a rant, which was easily long enough to last through any medical appointment or interview, and he was able to keep up the facade of polite socially acceptable behaviour.

After both nursing home interviews, Fulton's polished veneer would soon fade away, and he would become exhausted by 'keeping up the façade' that everything was okay, and would quickly regress into his Dementia behaviours, when alone with me.

He did have an Aged Care Assessment Team (ACAT) assessment which confirmed where he was on the Dementia scale.

I think his good presentation may have impressed both the doctors and the nurse manager enough to ascertain he really was low care, not high care as his testing showed him to be. What was wrong with that? Just like a little boy presenting to the principal at a new school, Fulton gave a good impression at both of his interviews.

I quickly learned that a high-level care Dementia patient is about as welcome to some respite care facilities (or nursing homes) as a bull in a China shop. No doubt this is due to the fact it takes more staff to care for them than a regular aged care patient – less profit! This fact may have led to his first expulsion.

But I am jumping ahead of myself. Prior to entering a nursing home, a vacancy for a week-long respite stay occurred soon afterwards and I was able to leave Fulton there, to go with Alycia on our planned trip to Victoria. However, our break from the Dementia journey was short-lived.

I was shocked when I received a call from the respite care manager who asked me to remove Fulton as soon as possible. 'You cannot possibly look after Fulton by yourself, we will arrange another ACAT assessment tomorrow.'

I was totally confused as they already knew Fulton was 'high care' when he had been placed there for a short four-day stay.

Alycia and I were upset by this news but at the same time I was relieved that professional nurses and care workers could not cope with his needs, as I had been struggling to manage him myself for over a year. My guilt at feeling I was failing Fulton as his wife and his carer abated somewhat when I realised professional nurses and care workers found him impossible to care for, even for just one night!

Along the journey nobody had explained to me what to expect. I just muddled along like in the *Finding Nemo* movie – to 'just keep swimming' (moving forward) – hoping everything would work out eventually.

So we returned to Canberra and my nursing home search began in earnest, as now I had received professional advice that Fulton needed to be placed in a nursing home catering to the needs of high-care Dementia residents.

Now I had to find the best permanent full-time nursing home for Fulton, but which one on my list was it to be? I had never even visited a nursing home, and had no prior knowledge of how they functioned.

I knew I had to research my choice thoroughly and methodically and record my reasons for making the final choice. When I had started any new project during my teaching career, I bought a notebook and labelled it appropriately, so now the label read *Nursing home choice*. Some may laugh at such an antiquated method of recording information. You may wish to do this on your computer or mobile. But I did what I was most comfortable with, using pen and paper. When I sat at our dining table to update my journal Fulton would tell me to 'stop working'!

Although my nursing home information-gathering chats with friends were carried out informally, often over a cuppa in a coffee shop or in their home, my recording of their advice was formal. As soon as I returned home, I would sit at the dining room table and record what I had been told that day.

Fulton would say, 'You are very busy today. You work too hard.'

I did not share with him all that I was doing, and as he could no longer read, I did not worry that the notes I made would upset him. My notebook proved invaluable over the ensuing months and eased my load considerably. I recorded details, contact addresses and anecdotal information.

All essential information gathered that related to Fulton was recorded within its pages. It helped the family from time to time if they needed to phone his doctor or book an appointment for me. It was all there in one place readily accessible to the family and myself.

My search had three distinct sources in the criteria information-gathering process. The first revolved around personal recommendation and anecdotal information gleaned from the stories of friends, neighbours and family who had placed a spouse or family member in care over the past five years. Some of the stories of neglect and abuse were hard to hear and heart breaking.

Sometimes a nursing home made my 'possible' list because of three or four glowing recommendations, only to be permanently removed by an equally horrific contradictory report.

Through my conversations with our home carers, who looked after Fulton for a few hours a day over the past year, they shared their contemporary knowledge of the best, most suitable and 'don't go near' nursing home options available.

Most of these carers had become very close to Fulton and myself, and wanted the best care for him too.

Of course they said, 'Ethically we cannot recommend a specific nursing home,' but often proceeded to give me anecdotal information on different homes they had worked at in the past, which I later recorded in my notebook. Their assistance in this project was invaluable as they often had first-hand insightful information of life for the patient inside the nursing home. Their information enabled me to formulate criteria on what defines a good nursing home.

Specifically, I learned which nursing homes provide a good ratio of nurses to residents, how many registered nurses were employed, how many care workers were employed, and what the meals were like. The provision of nutritious meals is also very important to the health of all nursing home residents.

The second part of this process involved visiting the three most highly recommended places which I had on my list. I did this in two ways. Firstly, by making an appointment with the manager to be given a guided tour of the home and an interview where Fulton's high care needs were always discussed.

At this stage a couple of the proposed places dropped out ... 'Oh he's high care, is he? Well, I am so sorry we have no high-care places available for 6 months ...' By that time, I knew Fulton would probably no longer be in need of a nursing home bed, due to his escalating physical deterioration.

The other way to complete a picture of how a specific home functioned was to pop in to 'visit' a patient. Then I could go unannounced and wander around checking out the status quo. Of course, I had to first find 'a real patient' to visit, sometimes the relative of a friend, so I could genuinely register at the front desk as a 'visitor'.

I endorse using any such method that works for you. I have never been the type of person who indulges in such secretive practices, but only last year I felt vindicated in doing this by a story I heard at an Alzheimer's workshop in Sydney. During the coffee session I chatted with an elderly lady who was accompanied by a younger woman. Apparently, her husband was in the final stages of Dementia and was living in a suburban nursing home in Sydney. She introduced me to the younger woman as her 'niece'. After I shared various experiences, I had in trying to find a good nursing home for Fulton, she confessed to me that she also had been concerned about the care her husband was receiving.

Her solution was very interesting. She employed this young woman, a qualified aged-care nurse, to visit her husband at various times during the week. Her reason for creating the 'niece' persona was so the nursing home staff would not feel threatened by regular 'visits' from a qualified nurse practitioner. At the same time the elderly lady felt the nurse may be able to check on any poor professional practice which she herself may not have noticed.

The nurse/niece told me she had worked for a number of years in a nursing home and said, 'I know what can happen sometimes through under-staffing. I feel happy I can alleviate Mrs x's concerns about her husband's care.'

He was non-verbal, could no longer recognise his wife of 50 years or any of his family members, so was vulnerable to possible abuse. The nurse care-worker told me she had done similar work for other concerned Dementia family carers for the past five years. She later confessed, 'This is the most rewarding job I have ever had.'

The third method I used to make my choice was 'gut instinct' or the 'feel' of a place. It is the sort of feeling you may get when buying a home. You just know when the place feels right.

After all my research I finally found the nursing home which impressed me at every level of my decision-making. Best of all, I instinctively liked the attitude of the manager, not only was she a thoroughly professional woman but she was empathetic in her manner. I was impressed by all the staff I met, both nurses and care-workers alike. So I decided then that this should be where Fulton would live permanently.

However, my thorough research in choosing this nursing home for Fulton, turned out to be a dismal failure at first. Why was this?

The nursing home I decided would be best for Fulton – and met all my criteria, plus it just felt right – I had ruled out initially on discovering a patient had been allegedly killed there by another patient! I was horrified to hear this. So I returned there to tell the manager I wished to remove Fulton's name from the waiting list. Nor was I prepared at that time to listen to any explanations the manager gave me about this incident or how, and why, it had occurred.

The local paper had covered the story on the front page, so I felt I knew enough to make my decision. I had thought, how horrible that one Dementia patient had allegedly killed his room-mate. How could that happen in a fully staffed, professionally run nursing home? Of course, I immediately thought that I would never let my husband live in a place like that!

So then I chose another nursing home for Fulton which was second on my original choice list. Unfortunately, he only lasted there one night – exactly repeating the bad experience that had occurred earlier in respite care.

A few months later, having no other place to turn to after Fulton was expelled from this first nursing home residence, I returned to talk to the manager again at the original nursing home where the death had occurred. Initially I had been most impressed when visiting this nursing home and felt this it could best cope with Fulton's needs. It was my own lack of knowledge about the nature of Dementia which had caused me to not understand what can happen in a high-care Dementia unit. A shockingly tragic event which can happen in any nursing home if there are not enough staff supervising patients at all times.

So my mistake initially was prejudging a nursing home on the basis of one shocking event and being swayed by attractive rooms and smiling staff at another home. I had not known to ask relevant questions such as:

- How are high-care patients kept safe?
- How many staff are on duty at night?
- Have there been any reported violent incidents lately?

My problem had been that I did not have sufficient knowledge about the day-to-day functioning of a nursing home housing high-care patients.

I did not realise that there are no locks on doors because 'that could be a fire hazard'. Consequently, any Dementia patient may become disoriented after using the toilet at night and wander back to the wrong room and hop into an already occupied bed! This of course can be terrifying for all concerned.

But when I made my original choice for Fulton, I assumed that patients would be fully supervised all night. An impossible task when the night ratio of staff to patient may be one to 50! Easy for one wandering patient not to be noticed ...

Now many nursing homes have cameras installed, but Dementia patients can still become disoriented and often have no conception of which is their own room. The best analogy I can think of is to imagine a toddler staying alone in a big motel kept in darkness at night with all the doors wide open. Once you get this picture you can imagine what may occur in a nursing home providing housing care for a number of high-needs Dementia patients.

Now you may be interested to hear what went wrong at the first nursing home where Fulton took up residence (second choice on my original list). The manager had shown me a lovely display room, pretty curtains hung at a large window overlooking an attractive garden, matching bedspread on which a handmade patchwork quilt was strategically draped across the foot of her bed. Tastefully upholstered chairs were placed invitingly for visitors, which I later learned belonged to her mother. A large TV was on one wall and silver framed family photos were displayed on a small cedar occasional table, while small pieces of bric-a-brac and books lay on the shelves.

'We encourage our residents to personalise their rooms,' she said sweetly. Now I know this is how a typical low-care unit looks. At that time, I was totally taken in by this presentation almost immediately, the whole place looked so attractive and 'homey'.

Best of all, I could not smell the immediate aroma of incontinence which permeated some of the other nursing homes, causing me to automatically remove them from my

shortlist in my note book. This stale smell of urine lingered in the hallways of most of the facilities I visited on my quest, which sometimes would hit me like a battering ram.
In hindsight this 'eau de wee parfum' was a key indicator that insufficient staff were employed to take care of patient hygiene needs. Some of the more expensive facilities were amongst offenders of this basic care principle.

So this nursing home I inspected passed all my tests with flying colours. This home just did not have that institutional depressingly clinical 'feel'. It appeared to have kind, friendly staff, so all the boxes were ticked. I was 'hooked' and Fulton also seemed happy on looking around on our initial inspection.

I had not taken him to look at all the nursing homes I visited, only the first two choices on my list.

After our inspection, I brought Fulton to meet the staff and have a look around. Fulton then was interviewed by the manager and we waited a few days to see if we could go ahead with our application. Fulton passed his interview, even though he had a high-care assessment, and the manager said the magic words, 'We have a vacancy.'

I could not believe our luck. Finally I had found what I thought to be the perfect nursing home for my husband. At last my search was over.

However, there was no happy ending. Despite all my thorough inspections, research, interviews and the right 'feel'. Fulton's first day at his new home ended shockingly and became his last day there.

But more of that later.

First, I had the pleasure of telling my children that night that I had found the perfect place. I witnessed their relief at hearing their father could go to a pleasant home and that I could have some rest.

The following day I went shopping. I bought a new TV, a comfortable adjustable leather chair for Fulton's room, and several pairs of pyjamas, slippers and a dressing gown. That night I spent hours sewing name labels on to every piece of his clothing in preparation for his move.

The next morning, Alycia helped Fulton and me to move him into his new home. She spent the first hour stomping on masses of 'imaginary ants' Fulton could see as he sat in his new chair. To distract him from the ants, I turned on the TV but he immediately put his hands over his eyes and shouted, 'They're coming to get me.'

The nurse popped her head around his door suggesting, 'Maybe you should leave now and let Fulton settle in.' She handed me an envelope and said, 'You need to fill this in for our records. Please bring it back as soon as possible.' She certainly offered no comforting words to me.

As I turned and left my husband in his new home, I was feeling very emotional as this was to be the last time we lived together, so heart-breaking after 40 years.

Alycia and I both felt unhappy at leaving Fulton there. When I went home, I opened the envelope. Inside was a form headed 'End of life plan' in which details of the funeral home to which Fulton should be moved after his death were to be completed. I realised then what I had known for months that Fulton would never come home again.

I had a real sense of foreboding as I fell asleep that night. My feelings were justified. The following morning I received an early call to say the facility was not suitable for him, 'There has been an incident!' and he must be removed immediately.

I thought, 'Not again.' You cannot even imagine my distress. What had happened? Where could he go now? After all the paperwork assessments, bank transfers, moving in of furniture and unpacking his belongings, they could not cope with his behaviours, not even for one night! Yet they knew he was 'high-care'. So what would I do now?

I knew that none of the other nursing homes suitable for high-care needs had immediate vacancies. These were the thoughts racing through my mind as I drove to the nursing home.

On my arrival there I found that Fulton had been transferred by ambulance to Canberra Hospital. So I then had to drive to the hospital, not really knowing what had happened. After a rather traumatic time in the emergency department, which involved Fulton wandering away, I thankfully found him in the ambulance bay, unsupervised, with not a hospital staff member in sight! I was shocked and did not know what to do next, nor were staff forthcoming with advice.

This situation was particularly stressful as I was unsure if Fulton had been injured, if he required medical attention, or if he had even received medical attention. I calmly put my arms around him, and slowly motioned him back into the emergency department, so that I could work out what on earth was going on at 8am in the morning! A short time later I was assertively instructed by staff that Fulton was to be discharged!

Unbelievable. Where to now? I despaired.

I began to understand the need for a Dementia liaison officer who could liaise and advocate specifically for Dementia patients, in a similar way that NDIS Health Liaison officers work, in a crisis situation like this, to support NDIS participants.

Had I not been with Fulton for the 24 hours in emergency, I do wonder what may have happened to him. Even with my presence, it was very difficult for me to find suitable on-going accommodation for him, especially as I had no knowledge of what facilities could be available across the Canberra health providers. The lack of a 'wrap-around' support for people with Dementia in crisis, and their carers/families across the Health and Aged Care systems in Canberra is alarming, to say the least.

Our problem was that Fulton, having been unexpectedly expelled and taken to the hospital, was about to be discharged from the emergency department at 9am on a Saturday morning with no placement he could go to. I felt totally abandoned by this systemic failure in the emergency discharge process.

Once a patient is discharged from a hospital, I found there was little or no advocacy, or advice, for people with Dementia and their carers. It seemed to me that the different health facilities providing health care services for the aged and adult mental health patients do not communicate with each other effectively or collaboratively. Let alone back to the carers of people with Dementia.

Apparently, there is a Dementia advocacy service in Canberra, but during my connection with the nursing home and aged care services, nobody told me of its existence. All the hospital staff I asked said it was not part of their job to find Fulton accommodation.

Fortunately, after hours on the phone, I was able to have him admitted to a special unit at another hospital for assessment. Fulton stayed there for treatment and evaluation for two weeks. This enabled me to find another nursing home placement.

It was an awful experience for me and terrifying for Fulton, who had less idea than me as to why he was being transported from one place to another. From the hospital he then went to an emergency respite care facility for two weeks. While he was there, I visited him daily. Each day I also continued calling other nursing homes to try to find a permanent place for him.

This experience was traumatic and emotionally draining. I thought, 'I just do not have the strength to keep battling on Fulton's behalf.' I cannot imagine what happens to patients having advanced Dementia whose partner is elderly or infirm. Who advocates for them then?

What was obvious was that very few nursing homes wanted to take another high-care patient.

But, at last, I was very fortunate in finding a vacancy had occurred at the nursing home I had originally rejected. After our nightmare experiences in the interim I had accumulated a great deal of understanding and knowledge about Dementia care. Now I realised how much the Dementia behaviours change as the symptoms escalate over time – and a previously calm, peaceful person may spontaneously exhibit totally new behaviour which can be potentially violent. Often the right approach may defuse a situation and an explosive outburst may be avoided.

What I had originally believed was that this nursing home must cater for the needs of patients who had developed a type of Dementia which Fulton did not have. Later, I realised it was professionally prepared to cater to all the needs of high-care Dementia patients, like Fulton had become.

After learning more about Dementia and experiencing Fulton's escalating Dementia-related behaviours, I now knew this nursing home had suitable facilities, activities and professionally trained staff to cater for the needs of all high-care Dementia patients.

Unfortunately, we learned through bad experiences that only certain nursing homes are equipped, and have the appropriately trained staff, to meet the needs of high-care Dementia patients.

I now learned that this original nursing home had been substantially updated in the interim since my first visit. All patients now had their own rooms. And cameras had been installed as an extra security measure.

Most of the problems which we experienced in finding a nursing home suitable for Fulton's needs were caused by the lack of information readily available to prospective patients concerning medical services offered within the health system. I was not told by Fulton's gerontologist that Fulton could gain admission to a special unit at a Canberra hospital for further assessment. There was so much I learned too late to help Fulton.

However, I was pleased that Fulton finally settled in so well with appropriate care – and support for the family was also provided. He lived there comfortably until his death five months later.

When Fulton moved to this final nursing home, I again tried to create a pleasant space. I wanted to make Fulton's room as comfortable as possible by having familiar family photos on the walls for him to look at when I was not there. But this time, as his room was in the high-care area of the facility, we were specifically told not to have anything that could be thrown in the room. Photos in frames were a 'no-no' as they could be thrown or used as a weapon. So no picture frames, vases or any personal effects were permitted!

This explains the rather utilitarian décor which initially I had felt was cold and unfriendly. I had thought the home presenting the cosy atmosphere preferable to this one. I knew now I was wrong in my initial judgement as it was not a good idea to have decorative items strewn about which the high-care patient could use as a weapon!

Our daughters did not realise this yet. So Alycia and Fiona copied some photos and laminated them so they could be stuck on any surface and would not hurt anyone if thrown at them! One of the nurses suggested kindly that we take them home, as other patients would most likely steal them.

We soon learned from the caring staff that the high-care patients all have very different behaviours from the low-care patients.

We had created a photo journal which had large A4 photos on each page depicting key events in Fulton's life, 'A story of my life'. We used this often to share and talk with him about family events, hoping to trigger a flicker of memory on Fulton's part. It was also handy to share when visitors arrived as Fulton was almost totally non-verbal by now. Showing them the album and sharing happy events with others could sometimes elicit a smile from him. We always took this album home every day, as it was too precious to lose or be torn apart.

The advice regarding the removal of framed photos and objects I received from staff, indicating that all high-level patients had a tendency towards violence, would have helped me a lot earlier if I could have prepared myself for the repercussions it caused.

Just as toddlers at kindergarten can suddenly 'kick off' and bite or hurt another child, keep in mind that any one of the fellow patients can also do so.

Again the family learned more about what behaviour to expect from Fulton as his condition deteriorated. The frustration and fear that Dementia patients must feel at not being able to communicate may often be expressed physically or verbally in socially inappropriate and scary ways. After a while, as a visitor you become used to the sudden shrieks or screams nearby which may be vocalised by otherwise docile patients. I was rather disconcerted by this during my early visits, but soon I became immune to these outbursts. Although Fulton had never been violent at home, I did witness a distinct change in personality as his symptoms escalated, when he was shut into the high-care area.

He often tried to do a 'runner' by silently following an unsuspecting visitor to the locked entrance and exit door. Access outside was gained by typing in a secret numerical code which Fulton did not know, or perhaps could not remember. A couple of times he almost made it to the outside corridor, by shadowing a departing visitor, only to be caught at the second door by a vigilant nurse!

Earlier, Fiona experienced her father's intention to leave the nursing home when she visited him one lunch hour. He told her to sit in a chair away from the table of patients with whom he was 'chatting'. She dutifully obliged but was concerned to hear her father say, 'If we're careful, tonight we should get a few out.'

She realised he was quoting lines from his favourite movie, *The Great Escape*, which he had watched frequently when he was still living at home. I guess I had not thought too clearly about choosing that particular film for him to watch. At the time I had had no intention of placing him into a nursing home.

Fiona was amused as she related this story to me. I always called a nurse to distract him when I was leaving. It reminded me so much of doing the same thing years earlier when Jon tried to escape from kindergarten when I left each day. His teacher would pick him up and take him outside to ride the bikes as I crept away. The guilt I felt on both occasions was palpable. Was I doing the right thing in leaving? Maybe I should stay longer?

The activities organised by the nursing home are indicative of the level of suitable care offered for all residents. Residents were usually seated in a circle in the communal living area, ready for the planned activities when the television would be turned off so the focus would be on the facilitator. Most residents in the high-care area would be sitting in their favourite chair, mainly dozing or quietly listening to the leader of the day's activities. I usually joined in each day to help engage Fulton in whatever was happening.

There seems to be a great variation between nursing homes as to the type of specialised activities offered. If you are in the process of choosing a nursing home, it may be worthwhile to check what type of activities are offered on a regular basis. This includes specific programs which have been developed by professional staff and streamlined to the needs of those residents in the high-care category.

Even when a patient is in the high-care stage, it is so important to ascertain there is some type of program offered to ensure the patient is not just left in bed or in a wheelchair all day.

At Fulton's nursing home there were a range of interesting activities offered. As Fulton had reached high-level care, many activities were outside his range of cognitive ability, so the choice for him was quite limited, but he was happy to sit and watch but did not participate.

Fulton was no longer able to travel in the mini-bus available for group outings as he was an escapee risk! But it was good to see the other residents regularly taken to the Art Gallery, the Botanical Gardens or for a picnic by the lake.

He was restricted to 'in-house' activities which I found challenging myself, as many were rather childish, like using play dough to make figurines. Although I did understand the reason behind involving the patients in these simple activities. When cognition has diminished, little can be achieved.

Exercises to music in a chair amused Fulton, mainly as he thought the other residents looked funny when they tried to kick a balloon around the circle. He had been athletic and had enjoyed playing tennis and golf only a few years ago, so perhaps found it humorous to be waving his hands in time with the music.

Once a week an elderly volunteer played an electric keyboard and sang old Vera Lynne songs to which Fulton's response on one occasion was a classic, 'Shoot me please' whispered loudly in my ear! However he did sometimes hum and tap his feet in time with the music. He had been Patron of the Canberra Symphony Orchestra and most likely would have really preferred some classical music or opera.

I read with relief recently that a program of classical music was being piloted by final year students from the ANU School of Music in one of the Canberra nursing homes. There is much that could be achieved by spending time and effort looking into what may help people with Dementia become engaged, calm and peaceful.

Although there were opportunities for Fulton to mix with the other residents he mainly preferred to sit alone in the garden, if the weather permitted. I frequently wheeled him outside to sit under the trees where he relaxed peacefully. I found the garden essential to my own wellbeing, as I found the inside area rather depressing and sometimes the aroma would take my breath away! I preferred the perfume of the flowers.

On the nursing home journey there are many ongoing costs. These may include the constant drain of having to purchase new clothes to replace those which have gone missing on the way to or from the laundry, or the neverending pharmaceutical and medical bills. I had to buy replacement items such as pyjamas, track suits and shoes on a regular basis. Who knows where they all went.

Fulton's best clothes disappeared in the first few weeks. He had always dressed well and I made sure I left an ensemble should we have an opportunity to go on an 'outing'. This disappeared completely but the cashmere jumper was returned from the laundry shrunk to child size. Yet he had never worn these 'good' clothes whilst in the nursing home.

I had specifically placed them in a hanging travel bag in his wardrobe for special occasion wear, with a big note to that effect hanging from the bag. All his clothes were labelled with his name, so when they went missing, I tried to find them in other resident's wardrobes or at the laundry. But most just disappeared, never to be seen again.

Sometimes I saw another resident wearing Fulton's pants or jackets. I know Jack's glasses and hearing aid were lost at different times. I even heard of false teeth being permanently lost. These losses cause distress to all and are a significant cost if they have to be replaced. But as Fulton's health deteriorated, I just did not care or complain about constantly having to buy new clothes. Priorities change.

Along with the many confronting incidents I witnessed, there were many humorous experiences along the way. I have always been a glass half-full person. Humour also played a significant role in my way of dealing with life in general.

One morning Fulton managed to borrow all the walkers, one at a time, from fellow residents who were engrossed in the weekly entertainer's musical performance. It was during this hour that the carers usually had their morning break, leaving only one staff member in charge. I thought it was funny in hindsight.

I received a call from the nursing home that morning. A rather worried nurse asked if I could come immediately as Fulton had taken everyone's walkers and put them in his room.

Apparently, he was blocking the entrance to his room and refusing entry to all in quite an authoritarian voice. I drove over there quickly to avert a difficult situation developing.

After some time, I was able to convince Fulton that it was okay for visitors to our home to have their 'bikes' returned if they promised not to ride indoors! He said, 'This is a madhouse. You would never let the children ride inside. Why are they allowed to do that here?'

Needless to say, during my negotiation with Fulton over this mindset, I came up with some sort of explanation which satisfied him. He was oblivious to the death stares he was receiving from the poor patients who had been without their walkers for some time. I was embarrassed by this behaviour but was comforted by the fact that nobody was hurt.

Had the situation been allowed to escalate, it may not have ended so well. I was grateful that the nurse contacted me to help defuse the standoff between Fulton and the people who wanted their walkers to be returned. She knew that aggressively confronting a high-care Dementia patient may cause behaviour to quickly escalate into a violent confrontation.

Although I was embarrassed, mortified and shocked by this situation, I was pleased I had successfully brought about a good outcome and that Fulton still trusted me. I had been able to negotiate a good outcome which the staff had been unable to bring about. However, as I had seen other patients behaving in an equally aggressive and inappropriate way, I knew it was the illness causing the confronting behaviour, not the person with Dementia being a bad person.

I felt so sorry for the other patients who were forced to sit stranded for a long time as their walkers had been confiscated by Fulton. But I did have a laugh later that day explaining what had happened to our children. 'Your father was in control and seemed to enjoy telling everyone to get out of his way. He had a look of triumph on his face as he stood guard at his bedroom door, preventing 12 or so walkers from being removed from his oversight.'

This was just one of the many examples that illustrates that moving a husband or any family member into care does not remove all the stresses that Dementia brings to the primary carer. They just become different. In a high-care Dementia area, as a visitor carer, you will experience and see things like this that you would not have thought possible. The collateral damage Dementia places on a spouse and family can seem like it is never ending.

What helped me to cope with Fulton's escalating behaviour changes was the amazing support and compassion the staff showed us at all times. It takes a very special person to take care of the vulnerable and frail residents with Dementia. Something challenging was happening constantly, and yet the staff maintained their calm and professional manner at all times. Caring for high-care Dementia patients can be a thankless task, but I certainly acknowledged their work on a regular basis and thanked both nurses and staff for all they did for Fulton and the other residents. Sometimes I took a small gift such as a bunch of flowers or some movie tickets as a small token of my appreciation.

I also nominated one very special nurse for an annual 'Nurse of the Year Award' as I felt she had carried out duties well beyond requirements. She was very grateful for our family's acknowledgement of her care of Fulton in our absence, and became tearful when I told her we had nominated her for the award. Unless you have been a full-time carer, I think it is hard to comprehend the tasks a nurse has to carry out every day in such a constantly challenging environment.

So after a few false starts, I had found a really wonderful nursing home for Fulton where he passed away peacefully a few months later. During the first couple of months at this nursing home I found the nurses and staff all worked with Fulton and the other high-care patients in a professional manner. In all my times visiting Fulton there, I did not see any behaviour indicating that the staff did not take their job very seriously and were also able to communicate with the patients and visitors in a friendly, sympathetic and caring way. Yet at the same time, I did witness a lot of challenging and socially inappropriate behaviour on a daily basis from some patients.

Fulton however seemed to have calmed down in this environment as he felt safe and secure. He was living in his own twilight reality, which we all found a bit difficult to switch into or out of as required.

One day he believed he was on a giant ocean liner, remembering perhaps a sea voyage he had completed many years before. He said to Liam, our six-year-old grandson who was visiting with Bianca his mother, 'Pop down to the next deck. You'll enjoy the pool there.' Fortunately Liam, with the wonderful insight children have just said, 'OK, Fulton.'

On another occasion Fulton looked out the window and commented, 'The boys (his sons now in their fifties) love this house. It's so good for them as there is a big garden here where they can play football all day.' He must have been momentarily back in London when his twin boys were about ten.

I had learned not to question these ruminations but to agree with whatever idea or memory he was sharing, and to encourage him to continue. I thought it was good that, although his memories of his past life were jumbled up, at least he enjoyed experiencing them and sharing some with me. The days passed quickly as I visited daily and was pleased to see he was calm.

Sometimes as I arrived, he would be wandering around the garden with a newly acquired 'lady friend'. Apparently they spent a lot of time together when I was not there with him. She carried a large wedding photo of herself and her husband, clutched in her hands constantly. Her husband and I often sat chatting and he told me he had been visiting her for a couple of years. Sadly, she did not recognise him and ignored him as if he was a stranger. It was sad to hear that, but we both agreed we were pleased to see our partners had made good friends with each other. Do not think this this type of bonding between Dementia patients is unusual, as the nurse manager had told me about this type of friendship and said it was quite common.

Also sadly, some spouse carers become very upset when they witness this type of friendship developing, feeling it is some type of betrayal of their marriage. It is not, of course, and it did not worry me at all. It is however just part of the tapestry of changing behaviours which your partner may manifest towards the end of their journey.

There were still some happy family times for us, as much as Dementia would allow, when we sat in Fulton's room chatting with him. One of the most memorable was our last Christmas together, when Fulton even managed a final farewell wave to some of his children via Skype.

By this stage, Fulton spent all day in an invalid chair as he could no longer walk, so there were no more inappropriate behaviours possible. He was content and no longer battled the fog surrounding his brain. All his energy had gone after a spell in hospital with pneumonia which caused a downhill spiral in his health. Soon afterwards he spoke only in whispers of unintelligible 'mumbo jumbo'.

Then Fulton became totally silent, sometimes his lips would move but he just was no longer capable of making any intelligible sounds. I realised then his struggle was over, he seemed at peace and was no longer angry at his non-responsive brain. Nor was he frightened, confused or anxious. He was now calm and fortunately recognised us all to the end, by squeezing our hands or smiling at us.

Shortly afterwards he appeared to escape into a twilight world, of blissful sub-consciousness. I believe he was drifting in and out of sleep as one does in the time of waking from a dream. His periods of wakefulness diminished to a few hours a day. He seemed to know when I was sitting beside him, as he would acknowledge my presence by squeezing my hand or sometimes opened his eyes and smiled.

His doctor and nurses had told me that Fulton was reaching the end of his journey. They told me he had reached the stage where palliative care should start. After all our struggles, this was a calm time for Fulton and myself, as we both had come to terms that his battle with Dementia was over. Occasionally he smiled, he could no longer speak or eat but did manage to communicate with all the family in different ways.

At last his Dementia journey had come peacefully to an end.

BLANCHE AND JACK'S STORY

Dear Jenny
I fully understand your guilt but take comfort, Jenny. This is the path for all Dementia carers. A carer cannot do it all ...

***

The veil of darkness that descended on our summer holidays in Europe in 2013 had still not entirely lifted, even though we had arrived home safely. Jack still continued to show awkward and cumbersome moments in making connections to his previously familiar home surrounds.

It seemed very unlikely the reality of his comfortable life of only four weeks ago could return. For instance, when I assisted Jack with his bedtime routine, I noticed some suspicious paranoia and wondered again if he was figuring out my identity. But nothing played out, as he was too overcome with extreme exhaustion and quickly fell asleep.

The next morning, he woke up naturally that proved he had slept well and his body clock had adjusted to his home time. Yet despite the general aura of contentment, his ability to move around the house was hesitant and he was unable to recognise the various rooms in our home. Jack's facial expression showed joy to see Maria's car pull up the driveway with our grandchildren, and this showed some promise.

Now that I had access for Dementia counselling support, I had learnt to be brave despite being gripped with fear. The best advice I had was to be in the present and to notice when ideas or behaviours were not based on reality. But to accept the behaviours, to be true for the person with Dementia, and it was best to stay calm. I applied the calmness rule that I had learnt. This approach stops the delusion from further escalating and momentum is lost as quickly as it begins.

Since our return I had already reached out to Jack's GP to have him admitted into hospital, as Jack's unpredictable behaviours were now getting frequent, and it was best to act now rather than be sorry later. I had made an appointment to see the GP so I could bring him up to date with Jack's delusional behaviours that began the minute we landed at the airport and continued to accelerate with little warning.

The frequency with which these episodes were being played out, as sensory experiences and real, was leaving him and those around him dangerously exhausted, and was affecting all our sleep.

I also had to plead with the GP, 'Please do not interpret my story as incorrect, because I was forced to create a story from little bits and pieces that occurred occasionally.'
The major concern was to address immediately his frequent hallucinations and falls.

The GP made arrangements to have Jack admitted into hospital and I informed him that I had already completed the nursing home processes and had to wait for a couple of days for a room to become vacant! I also requested the GP to make arrangements for Jack to be transferred to the nursing home using hospital transport, as it was too tricky to do it on my own while driving.

Thankfully Jack's GP supported my request to have Jack admitted into hospital and he organised an ambulance to pick Jack up from his surgery. The GP gently advised him that a short hospital stay had been arranged, to carry out further tests, and the tests would determine the cause of his frequent falls. Jack accepted the GP's reasonable request, and he stayed at the hospital until his nursing home placement offer was confirmed.

A tip for carers: no person is equipped to handle on one's own the on-going emotional and physical load that Dementia throws for such long periods of time. It is important to seek help from family or health professionals immediately.

In addition, every person is different and so is the way they handle a nursing home transition. Jack and I often confronted our own deaths with a robust dialogue, long before he was actually struck with Dementia. Jack always optimised quality of life as his main goal or in tandem with curative treatment. He had full trust that his family would deliver the best option to meet his needs.

Even now I feel the intense pain that Jack was not involved in deciding his nursing home choice. If Jack had been diagnosed with cancer or a heart condition then we would have jointly decided on the process and would have weighed up the treatment options in a calm and supportive way. In this case, our family had to no choice as we saw Jack's decline and he was in no position to discuss any options or solutions for his care.

The hospital's social worker and counsellor checked if I needed help to adjust to our forced separation. But as Jack's advocate, along with the help of our daughters, I decided any further intervention would only add undue stress, rather than a positive benefit for either Jack or our family.

Prior to the move I had sought Jenny's advice as I found the finality of the decision to place Jack into full-time care very confronting. Jenny explained, 'I don't think anybody knows how hard it is to understand this grief, unless you have gone through it yourself.' She brought to my immediate consciousness that grief was too big to hold on one's own without sharing. She added, 'When I placed my husband Fulton into the nursing home, I too felt alone and unable to grieve, as our society and culture still hold on to strong traditions that when a loved one is placed in a nursing home it is seen as somehow wrong.'

Jenny said, 'I am meant to appear strong for Fulton and my family, and I can if Fulton is cared for by trained staff.' She continued, 'Society fails Dementia carers, as it does not see the intense physical and emotional responses experienced by carers for years.'

Looking back, it was Jenny, a carer herself, who came to my aid and mitigated my grief, with her ready support and listening ear. During one of our nightly debriefs, Jenny informed me, 'I fully understand and share your grief, as I have also walked the same Dementia path.'

Her unique approach helped me feel I belonged. With Jenny acknowledging my grief, she unknowingly laid the foundation that enabled me to accept the next level of the Dementia care was the right choice.

Even today, our society sees bereavement and mourning as being only acceptable once death happens. But Jenny and I discussed our forced separation when we placed our husbands into nursing homes as death itself! Seldom does anyone come forward at this time to ask, 'How are you coping?' or to send messages of support to brighten the day.

On hearing the Dementia diagnosis news, Jeannette came to Sydney and we started our search for a nursing home long before it was required. I had little knowledge on nursing homes and this had an added benefit because we had done a little homework before it was really required. This early planning also gave Jeannette the satisfaction that she had played a part in contributing to her father's care and, for me, relief that I had little glimpses to know what was around before I made my choice.

At various points, I felt very fortunate when I could count on our adult children's help to provide the much-needed support a carer craves, especially when tough decisions had to be made in a hurry. Although carers are regularly confronted with overwhelming Dementia symptoms, many wait until the situation reaches an emergency point. On reflection, to assign time to get an idea on nursing home choices, soon after the Dementia diagnosis was delivered, was the right move and the right time!

We started our nursing home search in the dark and everything was a blur, as I had no prior experience with aged relatives or friends. There were no official or independent guidelines published that we could use for comparison. For an untrained and inexperienced carer's eye, all the nursing homes looked similar. I found it difficult to separate the good from the bad, despite the frequent tales of elder abuse reported by the media.

To ease our search, we decided to make the location of Maria's home the prime focus for our search. With two young children, I thought it would make Maria's visits to her father less stressful. However, my idea was unacceptable to her and she may have felt too much pressure, with Jeannette in London not included in any specific care plans assigned to visit her father and free to come and go, in keeping alignment with her work–life balance.

My prime focus was Jack's care, so I made sure the nursing home was easy to access from where I lived, with ease of parking. With my respite care experience, I had learnt to 'respect' the carers who provided care in the nursing home, who smiled and showed empathy when they introduced themselves and, importantly, how they approached Jack.

I found most of the nurses actually do love their jobs. If not, it seems unimaginable to put on a happy face each day, especially when some residents totally refuse to respond to kindness. The respite care facility where Jack had a short stay gave me enough experience to know what to look for in a nursing home to be considered appropriate. Despite Jack's positive experience, he would not readily agree to go anywhere. He was only happy when he was home.

This short respite stay experience taught me to pay close attention to how the staff at a nursing home communicated with the other residents in their care, how they welcomed family and friends. The values and beliefs they displayed were the important markers and highlighted their priorities. With this awareness, I stopped observing the structures and surrounds of the nursing home as they no longer contributed to what made a good home. Even the well-established garden at the respite care centre did not entice Jack to walk through the beautiful landscaped gardens and be part of nature.

So I began my nursing home search with an open mind and discarded any fixed ideas that I may have previously harboured.

Jeannette and I visited three nursing homes that day. All were similar in their design. We noticed some residents sat idly scattered around tables, some stared into space, yet some enjoyed their solitude by reading, others worked on puzzles, whilst still others felt content to just flip through pages of the newspaper and magazines, and many were content to doze off in front of a television. The TV was always on as a background noise. The nursing homes also housed some fit and able residents who walked laps around the nursing home and, when tired, had their metal frames for support.

These three nursing homes we visited that day were all considered to be 'full lock-up facilities'. Jack had been diagnosed with Dementia, which I understood meant memory impairment, language and thinking.

At the time of my nursing home search, I had no awareness that nursing homes had different levels of care. 'High-care' patients were often housed in full lock-up facilities and it did not click that it could be possible that Jack could need such a service one day. Jack began his stay in a low-care unit, and I was not aware he could move to different levels of care when the time arrived and he needed extra support. I was happy when Jack was placed in a low-care unit, as he still had 24-hour surveillance cameras operating to keep him safe.

The final nursing home I chose came through by a random stroke of good luck! In 2013 I attended an Alzheimer's conference in Sydney that was open to all interested people in the community to provide information and a better understanding of Dementia matters.

Never did I expect to ever come home with a fully endorsed nursing home placement! What's more, the nursing home came with high and glowing recommendations from a past carer who had shared her very positive experience with little hesitation, as her husband resided at this nursing home for three years.

This woman approached me during our recess break, and enquired, 'Why are you attending this conference?'

I replied, 'My husband has recently been diagnosed with Dementia and I am keen to learn and understand the disease, as I have little knowledge.'

She then went on to say that her husband, who had been a GP in the country, had also succumbed to Dementia and had recently passed away.

I was curious to learn about her nursing home experiences, as I still did not feel totally confident in making a choice.

The recent bad publicity that was being reported daily by the media on elder abuse in nursing homes was creating this doubt. The little research I took into nursing homes was getting murky as I wasn't quite clear on what constitutes essentially a good home.

I said, 'Please tell me about your nursing home experience. Were you happy with your choice and subsequently the care your husband received? And on what criteria did you base your choice?'

I did not need words. Her facial expression said it all. Then she explained, 'The three years my husband resided at the nursing home, it was sheer joy and was stress free. It was a pleasure to visit him each morning and to see him content as his everyday needs were the central focus of the caring staff.'

She said she noticed that the other residents also appeared relaxed and content. She had full praise for the care provided by the management, staff and the carers, and talked at length about the clean surrounds, the spacious dining room and their tasty and healthy meals. She added, 'Although my husband was unable to speak, I sensed his comfort as he always appeared relaxed and content. The focused caring was obvious, especially when the staff and residents were happily engaged in their daily activities when I entered each morning.'

She continued, 'If I ever expressed concern, the staff were quick to act upon with a follow-up and, when faults were detected and brought to the management's attention, and if reasonable, changes were made immediately.'

Naturally, I was extremely pleased the nursing home in question ticked very box on my search list – and, the cherry on the pie, it happened to be in the area that I was looking for my new home! First, I had to sell our home, to get the cash to pay the bond fee before a bed could be confirmed.

Without hesitation and with the nursing home details in hand, I immediately made an appointment to see first-hand the home that came with such high recommendations, based on her years of experience.

When I entered the foyer, the receptionist at the front desk was very welcoming and her friendly approach only further reinforced my confidence.

Although I was not a local, it was enough proof to validate my application, as I was looking to move to the area as soon as I had found appropriate accommodation.

When I was taken on a guided tour, I noticed the nursing home was undergoing major renovations and would soon have two new lifts with ample space for the resident's walkers. This nursing home was central with modern city living and designed to meet the specific needs of the aged residents the facility housed.

After I received the nursing home confirmation letter, I had to arrange another meeting with the nursing home's administrator who explained the entry process and I completed and signed several house-keeping papers.

In hindsight, the glowing recommendations I received from a past Dementia carer simplified and eased my nursing home search. I was again lucky, as her opinion could have proved drastically wrong, as the nursing home was under new management with renewed policies.

However I made no further nursing home checks, as I was pleased with the reception I received and the amenities that I had seen were first class and sparkling, being just renovated.

Indeed, I felt lucky that I had bumped into this past carer at the conference.

Although the nursing home fell into my lap, I still found it difficult to make sense of all the complex and difficult administrative papers that had to be completed. It was an intricate and convoluted business to understand and make sense of them for an inexperienced user of the nursing home system.

The administrative side of the business was difficult to understand, time consuming, and as nerve racking as trying to get an early Dementia diagnosis. However to complete the entry process did not take years as the diagnosis had.

In addition there were Centrelink application forms to complete – that were even more challenging to make sense of on my own. Our income stream and all our assets had to be calculated to work out the bond fee I would need to pay. When you calculate all the costs involved for such care, it is indeed nerve wracking. The bond is held and that money did not work for us for all the time Jack was a resident at the nursing home. Besides that, there were the monthly nursing fees, medical bills, dentist, podiatry, private health insurance, pharmacy, hairdressing and other miscellaneous expenses to consider. The costs became a nightmare that I juggled as we had not planned to run two homes separately.

Furthermore, the nursing home bond fee arrangements can change frequently. My friend Jenny and Fulton had entered the nursing home only six months earlier and had different bond fee requirements, when compared to Jack and me.

This was nothing to do with living in NSW versus living in the ACT. Rather, the nursing home bond fee requirements had been changed by the Federal government between Fulton's passing and Jack's entrance into his nursing home. Luckily, we had a financial planner who was well informed on aged care policy and systems, and assisted in preparing the Centrelink application forms.

Although the nursing home administrator did explain the process well, it could be the tiredness of a carer and also unfamiliarity that make it difficult to make sense of the nursing home process. Jack was still living at home and I did not have enough time to sieve through the endless documents with a fine-tooth comb that this job required.

In hindsight, I wish I had asked some more questions. But in my confusion, and with my limited understanding of how nursing homes ran, I was unable to formulate the necessary questions. So make sure you have answers for the following questions:

- What are the nursing home policies and who develops the procedures?
- Who decides when it is time to improve the structures of the nursing home?
- What are the security arrangements in place? For example, how often in a day is a roll call taken?
- What training arrangement are in place for all care workers? For example, infection control, etc.

- Are there daily activities and recreational programs for residents?
- What are the ratios for carers and nurses to residents for day and night duties?

Now I realise that there are many other factors to consider when making a nursing home decision, including changes to government funding, the quality of management, along with the trained/untrained staff who each bring their own unique values and attitudes to the job.

But luckily the nursing home I chose was still well-managed and can also be said, I went into the nursing home decision-making with a mature judgement based on the experience of another carer, who had adopted a positive attitude and chose not to embrace a bleak point of view on ageing and Dementia.

In spite of our family's effort to ease Jack's move into a nursing home with diligent thought and time, we still collectively experienced pain and anguish witnessing Jack's physical decline each day, his on-going memory loss, along with his loss of dignity and independence. It led us as a family to come to the realisation that supported care at home had reached a danger point, and it was no longer safe to continue with home care. Nor was it easy for our children to accept the family unit had changed forever. And our marriage had ended, even though Jack was still alive.

Sadly, no one mourns with you. I found myself alone, but luckily Jenny came to my rescue with her support and guidance, as she and her family had already experienced our pain. Jenny acknowledged my grief and spared me the pain of repeating the frustrating mistakes Jenny had made as she put it, 'due to her ignorance of the disease'.

When Jack entered the nursing home, he was admitted as a low-care resident. It was the ACAT assessment report that the unit's registered nurse takes into account and the basis of care is decided by the ACAT report.

Jack stayed in the low-care unit for 18 months. He was encouraged to stay independent as long as possible, although limited care staff were on standby to give extra assistance if required with everyday tasks like showering, laundry and cleaning.

The family helped Jack ease into his new living arrangements. We brought familiar items from home that were meaningful. In the past, Jack enjoyed the power of music, and somehow it still continued to have a special hit in his brain. When he heard his favourite CD collection, he felt relaxed. I bought a CD player and the family enjoyed listening with him as it took us to the happy places we shared. We tried to arrange his bedroom in a similar fashion to the way it was at home, by arranging pictures on the wall, organising his favourite armchair to be delivered to the nursing home, his bedspread, and radio. He had a family photo album to flip through. I hoped all of this gave him a sense of comfort and security.

In the first month of being a resident, the nursing home arranged assessment services for physiotherapy, occupational health and safety, and a team of geriatricians monitored Jack's Dementia health. We also had to find a local GP, who was extremely attentive to Jack's care and was easily available to the family if we had any concerns.

The approach was holistic, as all staff were trained to engage with the residents in a gentle, caring and sensitive way.

The staff familiarised themselves with Jack's background, hobbies and interests, and this interaction allowed them to design activities that were customised to Jack's remaining abilities and aligned with his interests.

Jack loved gardening, so the nursing home had garden boxes built so he could stand and feel the soil run through his fingers. He planted seedlings and was encouraged to water and see them grow. Sometimes he sat in the group 'sing-a-long' program, singing old songs from the past. Yet he was quick to escape when he saw me enter and he was also free to opt out when his interest wavered.

He never formed friendship or responded to any of the activities on his own accord. Generally he was just happy to sit and watch, unless encouraged to join in. In the beginning, he enjoyed going on a bus ride but later refused to go when he realised the visits were the same each week! At least it can be said that he tried to be part of the team.

All activities delivered by the diversional therapist were specially designed to encourage residents to participate in practical ways through their well-planned recreational programs, like painting, flower arranging and cooking.

These activities I was told also enabled residents to develop close engagement with the other residents, and the activities enhanced the resident's moods. When behavioural issues occurred, the trained Dementia staff were able to de-escalate the issues without using restraints or medication.

After speaking to the diversional therapist, I learnt neurological behaviour is often caused when a resident is unable to communicate their pain or is emotionally unwell. These group activities also enabled the diversional staff to keep a watchful eye on each of the resident's health. The recreational staff alerted the medical staff if they noticed any visible struggle or discomfort whilst on recreational therapy, and this was later investigated by care staff.

Having placed Jack into an excellent nursing home, I fully endorse nursing homes as being very important for Dementia carers. Not only did the nursing home make a difference to Jack's life, but it also enabled me and our family to continue to live our own lives.

I felt comfortable coming into the nursing home each day and seeing the positive care Jack received and I enjoyed the daily interactions with the caring staff, the other residents and sometimes shared our stories with other carers who had loved ones in the home.

Jack also had access to monthly meetings with a team of psycho-geriatricians. The aim of the team was to avoid behavioural issues and prevent hospital admission. When a resident exhibited signs of psychosis, the nursing home staff were well-equipped and trained to manage the issue in-house. The unit nurse manager made sure I was given plenty of notice to attend the specialist consultation visits they delivered in-house and I was always present when Jack had his consultation with the team, and I helped the medical team if Jack struggled to remember.

Management made it possible for their residents to have such specialist care delivered at the nursing home, rather than being cared for in an unfamiliar hospital environment, where untrained Dementia carers do not have the time to cope with Dementia patients when they had difficulty understanding what was required and hospital efficiency was severely delayed. I found this service very useful.

Jack once experienced a short hospital stay to get treatment for pneumonia, and he struggled to receive proper care, as the hospital nurses were unable to communicate appropriately with Dementia care in mind. Jack's experience resulted in unacceptable behaviours and a deterioration in his clinical diagnosis. I stayed with him during the day to reduce the confusion and distress, as he could not understand why he was at a hospital and did not like being cared for by strangers in an unfamiliar environment.

The healthcare system at most hospitals faces huge challenges when they have to deal with the demands of increasing Dementia. The numbers are on the increase and proper Dementia training is lacking. While hospital nurses are medical professionals, their Dementia training is limited and they are often unable to respond appropriately to behavioural and psychological symptoms that Dementia patients display when faced with unfamiliar surrounds, staff or they cannot express their discomfort or pain.

With this negative experience, I decided that this was the last time I would approve Jack receiving hospital treatment.

After a few months of Jack's stay at the nursing home, it became the first in NSW to adopt the Montessori approach of caregiving. The Montessori method of education was creative and based on residents continuing to use their abilities that still remained intact.

The aim of the program was to give support to the residents in their care and for the staff to rediscover the person behind the Dementia, by getting to know their history, family, interests and abilities.

The programs were then designed accordingly to use the activities that remained, to further develop residents' strength with the intention to help, maintain and improve the way they lived their remaining days.

The staff also used language that focused on their residents' abilities and not their deficits, which helped the residents stay positively and meaningfully engaged, and gave them a sense of self-worth.

Another helpful and useful point I recall, the nursing home also catered for language and cultural diversity if required. As English was Jack's second language, he started experiencing language difficulties in his word choice. The nursing home placed Dutch language signs appropriately around his room and he also had a Dutch chart with questions, which the staff flashed when he did not respond to their questions in English.

When the nursing home employed a German occupational therapist, I asked him to speak German to see if he could get a response from Jack. I was told that when he spoke German, Jack turned around startled, and although he did not respond, he followed the instructions. I do not know if Jack had lost his ability to speak or if he could not make sense of any languages.

I also noticed in time his voice had become extremely soft and his conversation made little sense, until one day he just stopped talking altogether.

However, the nursing home did not provide a multicultural menu per se. For over four decades we lived together, Jack refused to eat pumpkin saying it was 'pig-food'. But when it was served to him at the nursing home, he ate with relish remarking that it was 'good stuff'!

I don't know with certainty if the Montessori approach catered for religious practices or spiritual beliefs. However, every Sunday morning a Christian religious service was offered to the residents and their families, and the chaplain and her team helped families and residents in their time of need. Jack was born a Catholic, but he called himself agnostic!

Although, I was no longer Jack's primary carer, I still had to figure out and learn the nursing home policies as I visited him every day – and became familiar with his daily activities – to understand the environment where he lived and where I spent several hours each day.

Even when mistakes were made, the management were quick to adopt a positive approach and acknowledged their errors gracefully. The staff patiently listened to family carers' grievances and changed if it was warranted. This made families feel comfortable that they were being heard and understood.

For instance, one year the staff went out of their way to arrange a private room for our family to celebrate Christmas Eve at the nursing home. This was Jack's final Christmas with us, and we cherish the lasting memories of that day, which was only made possible by the thoughtful and caring management and staff.

It took Jack a very long time to settle in his new home and he struggled to accept his stay at the nursing home. It distressed me greatly to leave without saying goodbye and I dared not turn around. Jack was still under the impression that he was receiving treatment and would one day return home and I played along with this game.

In the early months of his stay at the nursing home, he would spend most of his waking hours engaged in plans to escape. He monitored the front door and reception desk like a hawk, and looked for an opportunity to run out without being noticed. His plans were well calculated.

The front door opened wide and it could easily let in or out several people at a time, and he would engage me in these plans as he needed a reliable chauffeur to drive him home once he escaped. He would say, 'I'll drive half-way and then you can then take over.' I didn't take his plans seriously, but nodded in agreement when an appropriate response was required.

One sunny fine day on a Friday afternoon, Jack saw his opportunity to leave and took it, when he noticed the front reception-desk was unattended. He was on a mission, and nothing was going to stop him when he had waited patiently for this opportunity for such a long time. He walked out of the nursing home without being noticed and headed in the direction of our friend's home, to check if I was there.

This nursing home also housed residents who lived independently, and some of the residents were free to come and go as they wished, as long as they made a note of their comings and goings in the register provided.

I was informed later by the nursing home staff that Jack could have walked out soon after his lunch. To this day I am unclear how long he wandered around the area, but it looks like it was a considerable time, as he was overcome by fatigue after several hours of walking. He collapsed only a few metres away from the nursing home, at a girl's school in the area.

It was the children's lunch break and the girls fortunately had noticed Jack's struggle at their school gate, exhausted. They ran to get help from the teacher on playground duty, who arranged for an ambulance to take him to the nearest hospital.

When I later visited the school to thank them for their care, I was told by the school staff that as Jack appeared clean and well-dressed, the staff had taken liberty to call an ambulance as they presumed he was not a homeless person!

I still wonder how Jack's stay would have ended, if he had lost his way and got lost or hit by a car. The nursing home was situated in a bustling Sydney area.

That evening when I arrived at the nursing home to assist with Jack's evening meal, I was stopped at the reception desk, and told that they had just taken a phone-call from a city hospital, who notified them that a patient was brought by ambulance, distressed and did not know where he was, but otherwise uninjured.

After the phone call from the hospital, the nursing home decided to take a roll call, and it was discovered Jack was the missing person. After this incident, roll calls became a regular feature after the residents' afternoon rest.

I volunteered to check the hospital and the nurse manager of the unit, who had just ended his shift for the day, kindly volunteered to drive me to the hospital to check if the gentleman was indeed Jack.

When we arrived at the hospital, the unit nurse manager dropped me at the main entrance gate and drove away! I found this gesture rather strange as I expected him to accompany me inside and check if the person was indeed one of their residents and if he was okay. After all, Jack was now under their 24-hour care for over a year.

I slowly continued to walk to the reception desk and noticed Jack waiting at reception. He stood up smiling on seeing me enter and gave a big sigh of relief.

I helped the hospital to document Jack's personal details, as he was unable to speak. We waited for the hospital doctor to complete his medical check before I was given a hospital discharge sheet. The hospital receptionist also organised hospital transport to take us both back to the nursing home, and I handed Jack over to the registered night nurse on duty.

I do not know how long it would be before the facility would have noticed that Jack was missing if the hospital had not made that call or I had not walked in at that same moment.

I could not help but entertain these negative thoughts. The next morning I waited for a call, to hear how Jack had settled and if he was displaying any symptoms of his ordeal of yesterday.

The nursing home had failed in their duty of care, as many of the residents in their care had memory issues and yet the management did not have clear strategies in place to ensure their residents were kept safe at all times.

However, I did not receive a call the next morning and I decided to wait for the morning rush to be over before I made a call to the registered nurse on duty. The nurse who took my call casually informed me that Jack had slept well and seemed happy, despite his recent incident, and he had just eaten a hearty breakfast.

No effort was made to acknowledge their mistake or thank me for delivering Jack safely back in their care. The incident happened on the weekend, and I had to wait to see the unit manager on Monday.

When I questioned the nurse manager how many roll calls happened each day to ensure their residents were safely in the confines of the nursing home, no precise answer was given. The most disconcerting and disturbing response I received from the unit manager was, 'The nursing home that houses Jack is not a full lock-up facility!'

If this episode had a different ending, I sometimes wonder what rights I had and how the case would have ended!

Jack's escape now brought my grief to the surface. I became gripped with fear and wondered how long before Jack saw his next opportunity to escape. I became very angry that I had let Jack down, as I could not believe that he was able to escape without being noticed from a place that boasted 24-hour surveillance.

The acute severity of the situation played out many different scary scenarios, and I failed to understand why the nursing home security had big gaps in their safety system. I fully understood that I could not change the situation but, as Jack's advocate, I requested changes to be made to their nursing home security policy to stop another escape from happening.

I am pleased to say changes were made with some urgency, and Jack started to wear a bracelet that had sensors that would set the alarm blazing to alert staff when Jack was within range of the exit doors. That gave staff enough time to stop him from reaching the main door.

Despite my negative reporting on the above incident, I have learnt that incidents like these are unavoidable, as all big nursing homes have their fair share of limitations. What was important at the time was that the management saw the current policy was inadequate – and addressed it and made changes to their security immediately!

Even after Jack's escape incident, I continued to maintain my positive social connections with the staff and the other families in the nursing home. The home was essentially run by good staff who were technically proficient.

Another incident happened when the nursing home made changes to their pharmacy provider. Unfortunately, the administrative staff failed to make the personal change to my pharmacy record, and I did not receive a pharmacy bill for a year.

On my part, I did not check why I had not received a pharmacy account, as I thought I had reached the safety net.

The unit manager was very supportive and accepted their error and volunteered to pay half of the bill and thus relieved my financial burden.

Sadly, the recent Covid 19 pandemic has highlighted some horrific stories and poor nursing home preparedness, largely due to shortages of well-trained staff and specific staff for Dementia care. There is also the lack of government resources especially noted in government-run nursing homes. Hearing such disturbing stories from the Aged Care Royal Commission's findings on the TV news is hugely daunting and so scary that I had to turn the sound off.

However, I largely had a positive association with the nursing home, and I could not relate to any of the aged care report findings to my experiences of nursing care.

The nursing home chaplain after some time decided to run a mindfulness discussion group on a weekly basis. The course ran for six weeks at the nursing home, to assist Dementia carers to adjust with their newfound loss, as the chaplain saw first-hand the daily stress a Dementia carer faced as compared to other forms of caring.

The mindfulness course encompassed training which taught carers to be in the present moment, to stay aware and to accept the events unfolding, and not to wish things were different. Rather, to take advantage of the carer's abilities, instead of focusing on what as carers we were unable to deliver.

Each week the chaplain introduced and discussed mindfulness strategies from the previous week, and that became our assignment for the next week's homework. The course took a shift from a caregiver role and instead gave carers that much-needed respite and time to focus on their own needs.

The chaplain discussed with the group how to learn, to practice and to apply different habits and ways to stay in the present moment. I found for the first time I was able to focus on my needs and have the support of other carers who had the same experiences as mine.

My aged care transition began smoothly as I was able to access Dementia resources available in the community and also get support from other carers who had completed their caring.

The magic formula that worked and made my nursing home experiences positive was, firstly, the staff were well trained and the executive management stayed focused, with human care being their priority. Secondly, I made it my business to be seen and engage with staff on a regular basis and to get to know them. I provided feedback, both negative and positive. I also let the staff know I was happy with the support and care Jack received daily.

After Jack completed 18 months of stay in the low-care unit of the nursing home, I was summoned to the office of the unit's nurse manager, who alerted me to Jack's further physical decline and the progress of the Dementia disease that was now taking hold. I was informed that Jack would be transferred immediately into high care. This unit is designed to keep all residents safe and supported – and supervised care was available on a 24-hour basis.

The high-care unit cared for residents who are in the later stages of Dementia or for those residents, like Jack, who had additional medical conditions, and who had started to experience severe difficulties with coordination that led to frequent falls.

The high care area was situated on a separate level of the nursing home. Nursing homes sometimes refer to these units as special care units, dementia wings, secure areas, memory loss units, or locked facilities units. It was unimportant how these units were named, but what was most important, that Jack could get the care he now required to keep him safe and to meet his evolving needs.

The family still had easy access for their daily visits. The full lock-up unit totally restricted Jack's daily movements, which he had previously enjoyed to the whole of the nursing home, but these new restrictions did not bother Jack any longer. Now he was still able to move around the spacious floor of this unit.

I saw the light and accepted that a locked door security policy was established at many nursing homes, with the sole purpose to keep all residents safe, and Jack had reached a point where he needed supervised care at all times.

Residents who are housed in a high-care unit are still kept active by care staff who engaged in activities according to the resident's remaining abilities, with extra care staff readily on hand. They kept the residents' minds active. By cutting up their food, they could still eat independently. They allowed the residents who were still able to walk to continue their walking around the spacious floor.

A few residents seemed content to face a blank wall transfixed. There were some women who had regressed to their past mothering roles and clutched their dolls and tended to them as if they were their babies again. Others repeatedly shouted, 'I want to go home!'

Our family formed a lasting relationship with the staff, and we engaged in the nursing home environment by rewarding the staff on special occasions with afternoon tea, or movie tickets at Christmas. I have had meals at the residents' dining room, and have also joined in their special events like Christmas and family BBQs.

After nine months had passed in the high-care unit, the family were again alerted to Jack's physical signs of further decline. The progressive loss of abilities is a natural process of the Dementia disease. Jack's body started the slow downward spiral – and he could not walk or hold his own glass any longer. I was again ushered in to see the unit manager who explained sensitively. I found it therapeutic to be able to speak with a nurse who fully understood what I was going through and this was indeed comforting.

She explained that Jack would now require more care and he would start the process of palliative care and the nurse manager organised a palliative care nurse. I was reminded gently that the focus of palliative care was to preserve pain-free comfort at all times.

Dementia is a chronic and life-limiting illness, and it would be the palliative care nurse's job to maintain Jack's final journey by relieving his discomfort or pain.

However the unit nurse manager was not able to predict at what pace the disease would proceed, or the exact timing of

Jack's final journey, nor could any of the medical team who were assigned to keep Jack pain-free and in comfort.

***

Jenny and Blanche's tips:
Nursing home

- Start researching for a nursing home as soon as the Dementia diagnosis is delivered.
- Develop a plan with your loved one while he or she is still able to participate that identifies their goals for future care.
- Plan for the future by ensuring the financial and legal issues for long-term care options are in place.
- Discuss the plan with family members so they can help as these documents are difficult to work out on one's own.
- Record all nursing home research in a notebook.
- Research thoroughly at least three nursing homes. Visit at different times of day. Put your name on the waiting list for a vacancy.
- Look beyond attractive décor and find out what amenities and services are provided for residents, especially those living with Dementia.
- Ask the manager to write down ratio of staff to patients, how many registered nurses are employed, how many staff are on duty at night.
- Ask what security arrangements are in place. Are cameras used in all rooms?
- Ask what infection control processes are implemented?
- Ask if all staff are trained and qualified to work in this sector?
- What Covid measures have been implemented to treat and isolate infected patients?

- Take room deodoriser and your favourite perfume on your visits as you probably will need them.
- Build a good relationship with the care staff and carers who can help to get you familiar with the new environment and how the facility operates. Early engagement with staff helps them to see the different needs of each of their residents in their care.
- Engage with staff and be friendly. Reward with a small gift occasionally if appropriate.
- As the primary carer, it is important you try to check daily on the level of care being provided. You may need to assume the role of advocate now, in conjunction to family care, support and love. Alternatively, arrange family members to visit at different times to give you a break.
- Take some respite care for yourself!
- Create a 'Journey of my life' photo journal of the person for whom you are caring.
- Label all clothing and personal items.

Chapter 4

Palliative care and the final journey

JENNY AND FULTON'S STORY

Dear Blanche
When the doctor said Fulton was entering the stage of his illness requiring palliative care, I was upset as I knew this was the end. Unexpectedly, it was a calm time for the family, as for Fulton his battle was over and he seemed totally at peace.

***

Dear Blanche
Last night, you asked me about Fulton's palliative care.

Although Jack may not be at that stage yet, I realise you want to know what is involved and what changes you may need to consider. This will help you learn what may be required to support you and Jack in his final days.

It seemed such a long time ago that Fulton died, but your question triggered a traumatic memory for me, of the helplessness I felt about his passing. I had tried every avenue I could to stop the accelerating impact of the disease.

When I said I would email you some ideas I had about what I could remember, to be honest, I was procrastinating to avoid even thinking about the last months of his life.

It was such a sad time for us all.

But on reflection I realised this time of his life was for the family far easier to live through, than any other time on his Dementia journey. Dying is such a confronting, personal but inevitable part of the Dementia journey. I needed time to think and to remember what had happened to us during the final months and weeks of Fulton's life.

I think discussing palliative care with the family and with the caring team in the nursing home may have been easier for me, than for you in handling this sensitive topic.

My children visited their father regularly and discussed, with me and each other, the deterioration they witnessed during each visit. They realised Fulton did not have much time left. I did not have to explain this to them.

However, with Jeanette living in London, and Maria being so caught up with her own work and such young children, your daughters may need to be specifically informed their father's condition has deteriorated and he has reached the final part of his journey.

Do you have any friends or perhaps Jack's family members in Holland who would like to visit him before he dies? Maybe it helps to reach closure if a final farewell can occur.

You asked me what is palliative care? No doubt you can read definitions about it online or in Alzheimer's Association publications. Palliative care occurs when a patient no longer needs medication to prolong life. It does not necessarily mean death is imminent, but that life is drawing to an end. I would say it is the care of a patient that focuses on providing comfort and pain relief, rather than medical intervention to try to prolong life.

If you or Jack have religious beliefs or spiritual needs, it is a time when you may find comfort in talking with a minister. Prayer may help you through the darkest hours of Jack's final days.

You need to think carefully about what Jack wanted for his end-of-life arrangements. In this regard families are all so different. You need to discuss this with your nurse carers and doctor, plus Jeanette and

Maria. Then your wishes for Jack's end of life should be written down in an 'End of life plan' so everyone knows, and should respect, your wishes. Remember Jack cannot communicate what he wants, so you have to become 'his voice'.

Will chat about this on our next call. Don't forget to ask the nursing home manager about this when you visit Jack today.
Love
Jenny

***

When Fulton reached the palliative care stage of his Dementia journey he appeared to finally be at peace. This helped me to cope with the fact he was dying. It seemed he had come to terms with Dementia and was no longer battling against its effects in his every waking moment.

Now I felt strangely numb and unemotional about what lay ahead. I guess the adrenaline just kept me functioning. For the last couple of years, I was on high alert and was stressed by Fulton's struggle with Dementia. Now it became possible to relax and spend hours just sitting with him in the nursing home.

We had no idea how long he would be with us like this, apparently sleeping for hours every day. Would his death come in hours, days or months?

Alycia and Olli had planned to visit family in Finland for Christmas but were concerned Fulton might die while they were so far away. Alycia did not want to leave if Fulton's death was imminent, but there was no way of finding out when this would happen. Despite questioning our doctor and the nurses, nobody could give us any indication as to how long Fulton would be with us. After much soul searching they decided to go, which was the best thing to do, as Fulton did not pass away for two more months. So they were able to enjoy a family Christmas in Finland and returned to Canberra a few weeks before Fulton died.

This is yet another example of the unpredictability of this illness.

Fulton had only been in the nursing home two months when he developed breathing difficulties and a high temperature. He was then transferred to hospital late one night where he was diagnosed with pneumonia. Unfortunately, the treatment he received was less than perfect, just as he had experienced a few months earlier. Possibly this may have been because the hospital medical staff were not familiar with the special needs of a non-verbal high-care Dementia patient with pneumonia.

Fulton's general health deteriorated considerably after this hospitalisation and, on his return, the nursing home manager told me that Fulton was entering a phase of his illness when palliative care would be implemented. I had heard the term before, but really did not have a complete understanding of what it meant. She gave me a brief outline of how his daily care would be changed to cope with his deteriorating physical health. He had entered the hospital as a walking patient, yet a few days later he returned to the nursing home only able to sit in a wheelchair.

I realised that Fulton was now entering the final stage of his journey. I realised death was no longer something that Fulton would experience sometime in the future, but was now imminent. Doctors and nurses always sidestepped my question, 'How long do you think Fulton has?' We never knew whether he would have weeks, months or years, with us.

The night I received the palliative care message from the nurse, I returned home and went onto the internet to try to gather more information about what to expect. During an earlier search I discovered Elisabeth Kubler Ross's book *Death and Dying*. Reading her book had helped me cope with Fulton's diagnosis of Dementia which I knew was a life-limiting illness.

The nurses, care workers and his doctor all diplomatically mentioned to me now that he was entering the time when palliative care would be implemented because his health decline had escalated rapidly after the bout of pneumonia and his hospital stay.

I was well prepared to cope with Fulton's death as we had a few years to come to prepare. That does not mean it was easier to cope with than a sudden death. He had gradually disappeared over a number of years, so at the end it was only his frail body which remained for us to care for.

There are many books currently available on the topic. It may be helpful to browse through some of these if you want to learn more about what palliative care involves.

Facing the death of a partner or close family member presents emotions and issues that are unique and personal. As a librarian I had been trained to research, so it is always the first thing I did and continue to do when I need to learn more about any topic.

Those fortunate enough to have a strong religious belief may not feel the need to seek out information or read about this topic. I am sure that having the support of the local priest, minister or church community will help you to traverse this part of the Dementia journey.

Alternatively, others may prefer to talk to doctors, family and friends to help them share this difficult time.

The most positive thing I can say about a Dementia diagnosis is that you usually have plenty of time to come to terms with the death of your family member who has the disease. After all, Dementia is commonly referred to as 'the long goodbye'.

Decisions about palliative care should be made months, even years, before a patient needs this type of care. It is much easier to make crucial plans for end-of-life care when death is not imminent.

In Fulton's situation, I had been requested to complete an 'End of life plan' as soon as he moved into the nursing home. You will need to make decisions about pain relief and what interventions you want to occur. It may be helpful to prepare a list of all family members and friends, so they may be contacted easily at the time of death. Fulton and I had discussed this with each other many years previously so I knew his wishes.

It is important to discuss specific end-of-life requests with your doctor and the nurse manager at the time when palliative care is implemented.

Death and how to care for the dying is a very personal and sensitive topic. I believe it is important to discuss all decisions with the family to involve everyone in these end-of-life important decisions. Hopefully you will have done this at the time of diagnosis. The staff can refer to your 'End of life plan' to ensure your wishes are adhered to during this time.

I had experienced the death of my own parents so had been involved in palliative care before. I had also read about the stages through which you pass when diagnosed with a life limiting illness: denial, anger, bargaining, depression and acceptance.

My family all passed through some of these stages during Fulton's illness, but he fought his illness right till the end when he developed pneumonia. Prior to this illness he was able to walk, speak and eat. However within days he became permanently bedridden, needed a specially prepared meal substitute, and made little sense when he tried to communicate.

At first he walked with the aid of crutches, but quickly moved into an invalid chair which became his permanent bed. Occasionally we tried a wheelchair so I could wheel him into the garden. He always enjoyed being outside the confines of his room in the fresh air, as I did too. Some of his friends visited then and it was really pleasant to all sit outside in the garden as the weather was warm at that time of year.

Sometimes being inside the nursing home with all its characteristic smells and sounds can be depressing and suffocating. Escaping out into the garden area, sitting in the sun under the boughs of a gigantic tree was where we both felt more comfortable than shut inside his room.

Wheeling him outside soon became impossible, as he kept slipping forward or sideways in his wheelchair because he had no muscle control. So from that time, he was confined indoors to an invalid chair which had the advantage of being on a slant backwards so Fulton could not fall forwards. He always looked comfortable in this chair, but it was difficult to witness a man, who had been proud of his athletic prowess in his younger days, reduced to being totally incapacitated.

He had to be hoisted in and out of bed to be placed in his special chair. He would then be wheeled out of his room into a lounge area for a few hours a day. He usually dozed or slept peacefully, and only woke up when I touched his hand and quietly spoke to him.

After a week or so he stayed all day in his room. It was obvious that he was drifting off and would leave us soon.

What was really noticeable to me at this stage was all his personal carers seemed to know he needed their special care and attention. I was very grateful to them for this, as no matter what time of day I popped in to spend time with him, one of the staff was with him, tending to his needs.

During these last weeks I saw him every day and organised the family members to visit in shifts, so he was never alone. I tried to arrange family and friends to come separately, as he tired easily and could not cope with lots of people talking around him.

The palliative care team all tried to ensure Fulton's dignity was maintained and he was treated gently and compassionately at all times. The nursing staff were wonderful to us all and ensured we had many private moments with Fulton, but would be available nearby to answer our many questions about his progress, or to look after his physical needs.

When Fulton first moved into full-time care in September, he ate normal meals which I cut up and he could place the food into his mouth and eat unaided. Within weeks he had to be spoon fed – but after pneumonia, the food prepared for him was like baby food. He then was given protein milk drinks to boost his nutrition.

Finally, he no longer ate his food intake with cutlery, but it was blended so he drank it through a straw. At this stage he had great difficulty swallowing. I was so scared he would choke to death when I was feeding him, so I let the nurses feed him.

During his final days he sometimes sucked on mini water ice blocks.

It was quite a quick decline during those final weeks of his life. Although we were all sad that Fulton had reached this stage so quickly, it was a relief to see that he had no pain or suffering, and appeared to be totally at peace. He had fought Dementia for so long but now it seemed the battle was over.

Fortunately we had discussed end-of-life decisions during our marriage, when we were both healthy, with no concept that death would come so soon to one of us, in such a cruel way.

Over the years this topic was brought up from time to time, such as when our own parents had died and more recently when friends passed away. Fulton, having a pragmatic approach to end-of-life decisions, often said things like, 'If I die suddenly, put me in the wheelbarrow and roll me into the dam!' We both laughed at that idea, but he had not been diagnosed then, so death was something which was a long way in the distance. Fulton had been quite religious as a young man and in the past few years attended church services quite regularly. So I knew he was joking when he made this outrageous request.

Fulton loved sailing and he rather liked the ancient Viking burial practice of being pushed out to sea at end of life. Well, that was not very practical either. I would have liked to honour these wishes, but it was not very sensible or legally possible for me to arrange this for him!

However he was quite clear in our previous conversations that he did not want any medical intervention to prolong his life, if he had no quality of life. Therefore, years later when I filled out the form marked 'End of life plan' for Fulton, I knew exactly what he wanted. It was confronting but fairly easy to do, as I knew what his wishes were.

If you are continuing to care for a Dementia patient till this end-of-life palliative care time is reached, you may feel it necessary to move the person you are caring for into a hospice, if you and your doctor feel this is appropriate.

I had seen the adverse effect on Fulton's health and wellbeing, of moving him into hospital during his bout of pneumonia. I was very upset this had occurred, especially as the hospital nursing staff seemed unable to cope very well with caring for a non-verbal Dementia patient with the same level of care and compassion as the nursing home staff had shown. So I definitely did not want him to be moved again. I knew he would not benefit from another trip in an ambulance. Nor did the family feel it would benefit Fulton in any way to move him to a hospice, especially considering the nursing home staff had made it clear they could take care of Fulton's palliative care needs in consultation with our doctor.

Moving to a hospice may need to be considered if you are caring for your family member in your home or the nursing home does not have the staff to provide a compassionate caring environment for end-of-life care.

Fulton had a private room, and the family and I were encouraged to stay with him for as long as we wanted. If your spouse is in a shared room, you may consider moving him or her to a hospice to ensure you have more privacy at this time, as I understand most hospices only have single rooms.

Our daughters had prepared a tape of Fulton's favourite music for him to listen to in the nursing home. His room regularly resounded with popular country and western songs belted out by Glenn Campbell, Frank Sinatra crooning 'I did it my way' or hours of classical music, as his taste in music was quite eclectic. The nurse carers and other visitors told me they really enjoyed Fulton's music, as we did when visiting him. Sometimes the shouts or screams of other patients were rather disturbing so I would just turn up the volume when this happened.

You need to make an effort to think of things which will comfort your spouse or family member – and yourself – when facing this final journey. It may be that massage or aromatherapy would be something to consider. We are all different so I certainly do not think I should be too prescriptive about suggesting what may provide comfort.

Fulton loved his music and we loved listening to it with him. He visibly relaxed when listening to his favourite CDs. Hearing is the last sense to go, so it is important to keep talking even when you think the person you are with is unconscious.

On the day Fulton passed away, one of his closest friends Bill popped in for a visit. Fiona and I were there with Fulton. He had not moved for an hour but was lying peacefully in his bed with his eyes closed. Bill, Fiona and I chatted for a while and I apologised to Bill about the gold cuff link which Fulton had promised him if he 'went' first. It was a funny mutual pact they had over the two cuff links they had been separately gifted for getting a hole in one at the golf club. Over the years they reminded each other from time to time that whoever died first would 'will' his cuff link to the other. The three of us were in the room when I told Bill I had looked in vain over the past weeks for Fulton's cuff link in order to give it to him.

Fiona said, 'Maybe Dad hid it with your pearls, Mum.'

At that statement, Fulton sat bolt upright in bed, it gave us all a shock. He said nothing and fell back onto his pillows. We all knew he was trying to tell us where he had put the cuff link.

He obviously could hear our chatter and summoned all his strength to try to tell us something about the cuff link. Sadly, he died a few hours later, without opening his eyes or uttering a sound. His favourite Scottish tunes happened to be playing on the tape. I like to think he passed away peacefully listening to one of his favourites, 'Scotland the Brave'.

What you or your family decide to do during this time will be right for you all. Just as this whole Dementia journey has been for us, this last part of the journey will be unique for you and your family.

I did have a rather funny experience a few years prior to Fulton's death. My close friend Shirley was in the hospice in Canberra. It is in a beautiful setting overlooking the lake. Each day I visited I would wheel her out to sit in the sun, and she would look across the lake and would reminisce about her childhood and early married life. She was quite calm and comfortable then. A few weeks later as her health deteriorated, she became permanently bedridden and was on high doses of morphine to alleviate the pain.

One morning I was sitting quietly by the bed, one of her granddaughters on the other side. There was a loud noise at the door which shattered the silence. It sounded like a person with severe breathing difficulties gasping for air and snorting near the doorway. As I turned to see where this sound was coming from, I saw a large animal like a camel looking in at us.

I got quite a fright. The llama, as it turned out to be, was being led by its trainer and was accompanied by a nurse. The nurse saw my look of absolute shock and fear, was I going mad?, and said, 'It's OK, Jenny, this is our special friend who comes to visit patients with his trainer. Would Shirley like to pat him?'

I looked across at Shirley who was asleep and then her granddaughter who looked as perplexed as I was. I said, 'No, thank you. Shirley might open her eyes and think she's died and gone to hell!'

It probably was not the most appropriate thing to say, especially as the hospice has a strong religious foundation, but I thought Shirley in her reverie may wake and think if the llama came any closer that she was looking at Cerberus the dog of the underworld. Cerberus is often referred to as the dog that guards the gates of Hades to prevent the dead from leaving the Underworld.

Shirley's granddaughter and I had a giggle about the visit and I know Shirley would have found it hilarious if she had been fully 'compos mentis'.

Later in the morning I went to find the nurse with the llama to apologise for my rather rude reaction, and saw him visiting inside another room. The patient was stroking him gently and everyone seemed very comfortable at the visit. I did think it was very kind of the llama's owner to be prepared to spend time volunteering to give comfort to the dying.

You see we all are so different in how we approach the end of life and what gives us comfort.

Nor can you learn how to cope with the death of a spouse from a book.

One good thing about Dementia is that quite rightly it is known as 'the long goodbye'. You do have time to come to terms with the fact that it is a life-limiting illness. Your family member may have many happy years ahead after diagnosis. Sadly, through loss of cognition and changes in behaviour, you will have lost your husband or partner years before he or she physically is no longer with you.

The man I married changed and disappeared forever years before he was finally diagnosed with Dementia. So when Fulton finally passed away, the family had come to terms with the idea of his death and parting years before. However, grieving for the loss of Fulton only really started after he finally passed away. Caring for my husband both when he was at home and in the nursing home filled my days and nights. I had no time to really grieve for him then and to think of what might have been, had he not been diagnosed with Dementia, as my life was continually orbiting his illness.

After he died, it was totally a different matter, as then I had the time to come to terms with the loss of my husband and to living alone.

Immediately after his death, the family came to my home to arrange his funeral. Although we were all very sad, I think we were all rather relieved his battle was over and he had passed away peacefully. My daughters pulled out the family albums and bags of photos from my sideboard cupboard as they put together a collage depicting the milestones of their father's life. At last, we were all able to put aside the tragedy of the last few years and instead focus on the wonderful, interesting and fabulous life Fulton had experienced before it was stolen from him by the onset of Dementia.

There were many hours of laughter and tears as they assembled appropriate photos so they could make a digital album of his life to share at his funeral service. As music had been so important to him selecting a playlist was also part of their efforts. I joined in to memorialise Fulton as he had been, prior to Dementia robbing us all of the person we had known best.

Those days passed in a tsunami of mixed emotions for me. I think I was running on the adrenaline which had powered my body for the past few years. Those days, the funeral and the weeks after have been partially erased from my memory by a multitude of family-related activities.

Weeks after the last visitor went home, I was totally alone with my thoughts for the first time in many years. I had revolved my life around Fulton by providing his daily care and had been totally subsumed by his Dementia-related needs. I had no time for myself or my needs.

What did I want to do with my life now I had it back?

It is quite common for the Dementia carer to be affected by a type of post-traumatic stress syndrome. Caring for a person with Dementia from the time of diagnosis till death gives the carer little time for self. Adrenaline powers your body to keep you moving forward, even when it seems impossible to do so.

Sometimes I felt like the blow-up clown at the Easter show, where people gain a prize for throwing a ball and, as it pops up, another ball knocks it over again. For years I had been on full alert, in survival mode. Now after Fulton's death I could relax at last. Now I no longer orbited his Dementia world but could have my own life back.

It took a long time for me to sit quietly and read a book and not flinch when the phone rang. I no longer anticipated that every call brought bad news about Fulton's health. I kept my mobile next to me at all times, and would subconsciously freeze when it rang, anticipating the bad news it always brought from the nursing home.

Now I could plan the days and months ahead to do things I wanted to do. It took a long time for me to realise that I no longer had to cope with Dementia-related issues. Now with friends and family I could have conversations about topics other than Dementia, nursing homes, caring ...

This does not mean I wanted to erase our shared Dementia journey. But now I learned to look forward to planning my own life. I could also take time to really grieve for our lost life, to remember our happy times together, and to mourn the loss of Fulton.

BLANCHE AND JACK'S STORY

Dear Jenny

Palliative care evokes sadness for all carers. At the same time, like you, it was a period of total peace, to see Jack relaxed. It was especially comforting to see the whole family by his bedside ...

***

Every new stage of the Dementia experience brought its own share of the prolonged grieving process to the fore. The grief experienced when Jack went into palliative care was more complicated than feeling just worried, stressed or sad. This time I was aware the end was nearing.

I had been worried and stressed when Jack was moved to the nursing home, but then I could easily manage my grief, as I was able to distract or shift my perspectives or activities.

Palliative care treatment is given to people living with a life-limiting illness – and care and support begins with the intention to keep the patient pain-free and comfortable. Nothing really could have prepared me to accept this hurdle, even though I had ample time to get ready to face the end, even though I was fully aware that death was an inevitable part of this disease.

The signs that death was near began with the obvious signs of Jack's considerable weight loss, the laborious effort required to eat and chew food, his increased daytime sleep, total loss of speech and sound, and his diminished alertness.

The grief of knowing that death was imminent made the physical response to this pain intense – and this pain was different as it was not easily mitigated.

To deal with this grief and to acknowledge and accept the situation, I am forever indebted to the team of Dementia experts who for years platformed and circulated valuable information to support and empower my understanding of Dementia, as the disease took years to progress.

In the meantime, I learnt to verbalise my feelings with the palliative care team who visited Jack daily and who made him comfortable during the dying process. The team additionally made time to support my processing of loss and they attentively heard my concerns. Nor did I get the feeling I was being pushed away or ignored.

Even to the end, the Dementia illness remained in constant opposition. Each and every Dementia experience is unique, the way it plays out varies from one person to the next. And that is the reason why the palliative care nurse or the medical team of professionals were unable to give me a forecast of the length of time that Jack would require palliative care.

The best advice I received from the palliative care nurse was to accept the situation calmly and let the process of dying unfold. The consequences that flowed from a palliative care situation were now defined and it was up to me to resolve the situation by living in the present and to accept the reality that I faced. Even though I was fully aware that Dementia is a chronic and life-limiting illness, it was still difficult to be confronted with the finality – and to accept readily the constant shifts in the progress of his Dementia.

Even harder was the fact that I now had to accept that the time had arrived to discuss Jack's care plan the family had woven together with the sensitivity such a decision required.

The palliative care team were ready to start. In Jack's case, that included his GP, the palliative care nurse and the interdisciplinary staff from the nursing home, like the occupational and physical therapists, chaplains and the dieticians.

Although palliative care can be provided in a variety of contexts, like hospitals and home settings, the choice for Jack was that he should receive his palliative care in the familiar nursing home – with the staff with whom he felt comfortable and who had cared for him for years, in the familiarity of his room.

With my years of nursing home experiences to fall back on, I would not hesitate to pick this service again. The care that Jack received was positive. Again, I felt totally supported with the palliative care policies in place at the nursing home.

A splash of light from the late afternoon sun lingered at the foot of Jack's bed. He had just ended his afternoon nap and he looked at the clock and his eyes fell shut again. He was unaware that I had entered his room.

Having ample time before my next meeting with the palliative care nurse, I began to personalise Jack's room where he had spent nine months with his familiar belongings. I scattered essential oil burners, scented candles and his beloved, soothing oboe music from his music collection.

The palliative care nurse assisted my grief by providing useful information and support on dying. Their advice helped me to have a better understanding of what to anticipate and how to respond to the end-of-life signs, as this was my first close experience with death. The useful advice I received helped me to stay calm.

I had little choice but to accept that Jack's brain would never be able to think or to do what he wished again. I briefly updated the staff about Jack's beliefs and the values he held, so the palliative nurse could understand the man behind the Dementia. I talked about Jack's philosophy on life and how he applied these principles to his daily way of living. He would often say, 'When I am no longer useful to society, I would like to go someplace where I would not be a burden to my family or society.'

The palliative care nurse stated, 'Some people do not want to talk about death, or are unable to grasp the inevitability of death. This denial is traditionally part of our western society and culture because there is not enough conversation happening in our society. And due to this ignorance, there are times when the end-of-life care can result in over-treatment, under-treatment, or other unnecessarily painful treatments.'

The nurse continued, 'Without a clearly written documented end-of-life care plan, many families invariably get it wrong one-third of the time, with the type of preferences they make for their loved ones in their final days.'

Together, our family had worked on the design for Jack's care plan. It clearly outlined his life preferences, that he would have expressed for his end-of-life choices if he was still able to clearly explain what he really wanted.

Our care plan had also clearly stated that no clinical medication. But at all times, Jack should receive medications for the relief of his pain and to manage his distressing symptoms! The family also stressed the importance of integrating the psychological and spiritual aspects of his care. Morphine was only to be administered to relieve pain, breathing and his overall final care comfort.

The 'Advance care plan' document had five sections:

- Personal contact details
- Cardio and resuscitation
- Artificial nutrition
- Use of antibiotics
- We specified that under no circumstances should Jack go to the hospital; and all pain management and comfort should be delivered at the nursing home only.

Jack and I in the past would have had many conservations about our treatment options in a medical emergency, and the choices we would make for medical and non-medical interventions.

Death to Jack was part of life – and we would not have chosen to significantly prolong the process of dying if he had no quality of life. For Jack, quality of life was his main goal and this mattered!

Any treatment he received had to respect these wishes. Jack specifically made a strong point to avoid all props, as he did not want to be made into a spectacle, long before he was actually struck with Dementia! He would no doubt see the care plan the family had decided on his behalf as a gift and he would have readily accepted the principles we had adopted – rather than a long drawn-out decline in a care facility.

This advance care plan no doubt would have had Jack's full approval, as it was based on his philosophy, beliefs and values – and how he had affirmed life and dying as a normal process before he was struck by the Dementia disease.

Jack was never uncomfortable talking about his death. In fact, he welcomed such debates readily and played the devil's advocate at times. Yet he too was not clear as to the specifics of his final farewell, but when pressed by the family, he would reply, 'Death is for the living.'

I was advised by the palliative care nurse that a care plan goes into action immediately when emergency signs are obvious. A clearly written advance care plan gives the health team the freedom to act according to the wishes of the family as stated therein. If Jack lived in a country that had a legislated euthanasia policy in place, he would have raised both hands. But at the same time, he would make sure that adequate safeguards were in place to prevent his wrongful death!

The palliative care nurse was very impressed with Jack's care plan and asked, 'Can I please use this Advance Care Plan as a template for other carers?'

I was indeed fortunate to have had the time to prepare and design a clear care plan, because as a Dementia carer I had years to think and to prepare Jack's end-of-life wishes. Despite the considerable time, the constant encouragement and supportive reminders from the head nurse of the nursing home made the task easier.

The design of a care plan is still tricky. Much thought has to be invested and attention paid to the details, as this is an important document, sometimes called a 'living will'.

Medication, medical equipment, and supplies related to Jack's final care were provided at no extra cost. I never received a bill as Jack's final medical care was covered 100% by Medicare.

After a year of daily visits and the stress of watching Jack slip away, I knew I needed a short break away to reflect on life without him. Again I found that the medical team avoided a direct answer when I asked them to provide me with an estimate as to how many weeks or months Jack had to live when he went into palliative care.

After experiencing first-hand for many months that Jack was safely and comfortably settled with daily personalised visits from the palliative team of experts, I decided to leave the country for a couple of weeks, and our daughter Maria became Jack's carer.

The care staff at the nursing home and the medical team also supported my taking a short break to visit my family in London.

Possibly on hindsight, they spared me the agony of experiencing the Dementia decline that had started both cognitively and functionally.

Jeannette had offered to buy my return ticket to London so I could spend time with her and her family, to relax from my caring duties, and possibly she wanted me to share her grief as she knew her father's end was in sight.

I also looked forward to it, and welcomed the idea of having a short break from the nursing home, and looked forward to spending the time being a carer for our two young grandchildren. It was enjoyable to immerse myself with innocent children, to momentarily be distracted and find the strength to cope with what lay ahead!

However before I even landed in London, Jack had reached a stage of semi-consciousness and had become unresponsive.

With Maria now the emergency contact in Sydney, she telephoned her sister Jeannette with the news that their father's condition had deteriorated and was serious. I was still in the air and had not yet landed in London.

After I had showered and had breakfast, Jeannette informed me, 'Mum, I have just bought five tickets to fly back to Australia at midday today!' She continued, 'I am so pleased that I can have this opportunity to be at dad's bedside to bid him farewell. I hope we can make it on time.'

Luckily, we made it to Sydney with plenty of time and the whole family was by his bedside, along with his four grandchildren, for three days on a 24-hour vigil.

The team of palliative care experts, who were assigned before I left for London, still visited Jack daily, to ensure he received pain-free and comfortable care.

The chaplain informed the family gently, 'Jack is still here, still in reach, despite the ravages of the Dementia disease and death nearing. He is still here with us and able to love and be loved.'

This was obvious to us as a family while we stood around his bed in his final days. He seemed calm and restful. It is not to be underestimated the simple things one does by the bedside of a loved one at this time. They can still be counted as being rewarding even though we had no idea if Jack could hear or if knew we were by his bedside.

We found being with him in his final days enormously rewarding. As Jack so succinctly put it, 'Death is about the living!' It helped and gave us comfort to hold hands, whilst we spoke gently, softly and assured him of our love. We found just being with him in his final hours was enough, even though we could not do any more for him.

We listened to Jack's favourite recorded music playing softly in the background. It invoked joy and sparked happy memories of our past life together. It was sad, yet a joy, to see our four grandchildren, ranging from seven to four years, lined by his bedside stricken with grief, holding tightly on to his right arm.

Even when Jack's family from Holland spoke to him via FaceTime in his final hours, he had a smile on his face when Alphons in his usual manner started reminiscing about their family life together and told him family jokes. Jack passed away calm, comfortable and peaceful to the end.

Devastating grief followed.

As a carer for a Dementia sufferer, there is no time for self-indulgence. The Dementia journey continued as I stayed immersed in the therapy of advocacy to arrange funeral plans, in spite of the grief of the ongoing loss, and in spite of the pain that Dementia brings.

But in a Covid 19 world, the consequences of not putting legal arrangements in place made some challenges. The disease strikes suddenly and often people are unprepared. That makes it more likely that people's wishes for the last stage of their life will not be properly realised. That can cause distress for the dying person, as well as increased stress for their families.

The task to complete a care plan document can get even more arduous when families are suddenly left to prepare and fulfil the end-of-life wishes for their loved ones of all ages in a pandemic world.

Like Dementia, Covid too does not discriminate.
We are seeing that Covid 19 is not only about age, race or social standing in society. Anyone can be struck by it.

With Covid health, the decline is sometimes unanticipated, speedy and in some cases the predictions grave. That leaves many families too grief-stricken to fully hear the advice that the medical team are unable to help their loved ones to survive, in certain cases in a pandemic.

The process of discussing medical care for the end-of-life in a Covid 19 world can be seen as mayhem – unlike Dementia, when families have had all the time to discuss the end-of-life care.

I have heard stories in the media where loved ones are in isolation and the care plan decisions are left to the doctors to carry through. And, in some cases, families have resorted to making the decision over the phone!

***

Jenny and Blanche's tips:
Palliative care

- Discuss an 'End of life plan' as soon possible.
- Ensure the care plan is ready long before your loved one is in palliative care.
- Hand the care plan to the palliative care nurse when the palliative care begins, as it goes into action immediately.
- Prepare a list of family friends and anyone you wish to be informed when death is imminent.
- Decide who you want to support you through this time.
- Find out if the nursing home can provide palliative care or if you will need to move the patient to a hospice.
- Count on being supported to meet the person's beliefs and values when receiving palliative care.
- Accept that the end journey and the time a person takes to give their last breath is different for each individual.
- Avoid taking a break – be it at home or overseas.

Chapter 5

Hindsight-itis

Reflections on Blanche's and Jennifer's Dementia carers journeys

JENNY'S STORY

Dear Blanche
For a long time my memories of caring for Fulton caused the tears to flow. Now, after a few years have passed, I can be more objective about remembering this challenging period in my life without bitterness.
I am committed in sharing my Dementia-caring knowledge with other carers, so that hopefully their caring experience can be a little easier than mine was.

***

It is important to remember that whilst a Dementia diagnosis is life-changing, it is not immediately life-ending. So after diagnosis you may have many years to enjoy the normal activities relating to family life and, hopefully, also have holidays and adventures together.

Dementia progresses from the initial stage, usually when a diagnosis is confirmed, and may take a long time to develop through the middle phase, until reaching the final chapter. Although there are treatments to help alleviate the various symptoms of Dementia, at the present time there is no cure.

But what helped me navigate through this challenging journey was hope. Hope that tomorrow would be a better day and that maybe a treatment would finally be found. Research is so important as I do believe, and certainly hope, a prevention or cure will be found.

One of the hardest things I have had to come to terms with, both during and after our Dementia journey, was that I did not always ask the 'right questions' of medical professionals. Mainly because I did not know what I needed to ask. Or to put it another way, I did not know what I needed to know in order to provide the best care for Fulton.

In hindsight, I realised the importance of carers sharing their stories with other carers. Through listening to these stories, you may learn what lies ahead. In a way, navigating the Dementia journey at present is like going on a bush walk in difficult terrain without a map. Although each person on the Dementia trail has a unique journey, there are many shared experiences which may help other carers to not repeat the same mistakes.

Unless you have walked in a Dementia-carer's footsteps, it is almost impossible to comprehend all that is involved in this journey. Certainly a different perspective needs to be developed as to how best to take care of people with Dementia, especially those in the high-care stage.

I believe that a person with Dementia should be kept in the family home as long as possible. I found Fulton's health deteriorated and his Dementia-related outbursts escalated when he moved into the nursing home.

Many of the confronting revelations from the Royal Commission into Aged Care illustrated there is so much that needs to be done to help improve the care of the aged, especially those with Dementia.

After caring for Fulton at home for two years and visiting him daily for many months in the high-care area of a nursing home, I learned a great deal about Dementia with Lewy Bodies, as well as how to best care for someone with this diagnosis.

The main way both family and institutional carers can improve the level of their patient care is to understand the nature of Dementia. The restraint and sedation of people with Dementia has been strongly disapproved of by the general community. However, until you really know what is involved in caring for the high-care needs of a Dementia patient, I think it is wrong to condemn these practices with blanket disapproval.

Fulton was never restrained nor sedated whilst he was living at home or in the nursing home. In fact, there were times when I was caring for him at home, when night after night he suffered from terrifying nightmares, I wished our doctor had suggested trialling a sedative. But that did not happen.

It is such a complex illness and requires a great deal of medical and practical knowledge to assess what is the best treatment for each individual with the illness. I have documented in our story what helped Fulton to keep calm and relaxed when I was caring for him. However it is just not realistic to believe any nursing home could possibly provide each patient the 'one-to-one' patient care that the 'at home' carer is capable of achieving.

So what can be done to improve the situation?

Certainly, ensuring there are enough staff on duty to care for the needs of all patients is of primary importance. When profit is the main concern of some nursing home providers, employing sufficient qualified staff should be also. Realistically, this one-to-one ratio, except when sleeping, is what most high-care patients ideally need. Unless you have walked this journey it is almost impossible to understand this.

When I started on my quest to find Fulton the best possible nursing home, I visited the high-care unit of a nursing home and was shocked by what I witnessed. I was momentarily traumatised at what I heard and had seen on my visit there. Patients were sitting immobile in invalid chairs, others crying or calling out non-stop. I was shown a large padded room for violent patients to use so they could calm down. It all seemed Dickensian and I incorrectly thought at that time that these appearances demonstrated 'poor practice'. How wrong I was.

This was because I did not know enough about the nature of Dementia with Lewy Bodies to properly assess the needs of a person having this type of Dementia. Nor did I understand the type of treatments provided by a facility catering for a number of high-level care patients with this disease.

Later, when I had learned more about the nature of Dementia, I understood why this was so. High-care Dementia patients can become fearful, anxious, scared, terrified and very violent in a split second. They can become agitated unexpectedly, and if a staff member is not nearby to intervene, the nearest person could be harmed. The other thing to be mindful of is that many other high-care patients can be in a frail physical state, may be immobilised sitting in an invalid chair, or only able to walk with the aid of a walker. So it is easy to see how vulnerable they can be to an unexpected assault from a fellow patient or carer.

Especially consider the impact of placing a number of these patients together in one enclosed area. After being exposed to the range of behaviours demonstrated by other patients, I realised just how vulnerable all nursing home patients can be.

It is also important to consider too that many high-care Dementia patients are cognitively impaired and may also be non-verbal. This makes them as vulnerable as a toddler – and just as unable to convey to their carers what is troubling them as a two-year-old child. Hence the numerous dummy spits or temper tantrums which characterise some Dementia patients.

Recently I read an article written by Annika Smethurst published in the *Daily Telegraph* on 20 June 2020. I was not surprised to learn that more than 1,000 older Australians living in nursing homes suffer abuse at the hands of other residents each week, and many cases are not reported. Also, shockingly, a KPMG report estimates there were over 52,600 incidents in nursing homes last year and more than 60% involved residents using unreasonable force against each other. More than 80% involved residents pushing, kicking, hitting, punching or burning each other.

One of the most frightening comments from this report is that nursing homes are currently not required to report such incidents if the alleged offender has a cognitive impairment.

So who protects these vulnerable people?

Sadly, in the nursing homes where Fulton had spent any time, family members of other residents often did not visit regularly. Sometimes family only visited on special days like Mothers and Fathers Day, birthdays, Easter and Christmas. When questioning the nurses as to the possible reason behind this type of often unintentional neglect, I was informed it was the belief that as the person with Dementia no longer recognised them, there was no point in visiting.

This is so wrong. I believe that a loved family member should be treated with compassion and care, by all the family whilst they are residing in a nursing home. Paying for residential care should not replace family visits. These visits should, where possible, be shared amongst your family and friends.

These visits should be at random times as then it is easy to report any bruises or unexplained anxiety or agitation which may occur when, for example, a particular staff member is on duty.

As I have stated frequently, Fulton was as vulnerable as a toddler once he became a high-care Dementia patient. Would anyone consider leaving their toddler in a motel to sleep at night with only other toddlers in residence with minimal supervision, leaving all the doors open? It really does make sense that high-care Dementia residents should not be able to wander at will around a high-care residence. Accidents to staff, residents and visitors may occur if maximum supervision is not available at all times.

So this is my one hope – that somebody in charge of addressing the recommendations of the Royal Commission will address the need to provide private rooms for high-care Dementia patients and have the rooms fitted with 'stable-style' half-doors, lockable from the outside.

This would enable staff to do the routine night check on patients through the top half of the door. Keeping the bottom half locked from the outside would prevent patients from wandering at night, or indeed, during the day.

This slight adjustment to nursing home building requirements – the installation of stable doors – would keep patients safe all night or when needed to be separated from other patients for their own safety. For example, when the patient becomes violent.

At present, some nursing homes do have a 'time out' room to separate patients who are agitated. However, these patients may escalate their Dementia-related behaviour if they feel they are locked up and cannot see outside the room. Again, half-doors would enable the patient to see out, but would prevent them from moving around the shared communal areas in an agitated or violent state of mind.

Despite suggesting this to appropriate senior health executives and staff on several occasions in the ACT, when Fulton was in the nursing home, I was informed such doors would not comply with present regulations as they are a fire hazard! Hopefully, this attitude will change soon – as many serious incidents could be averted.

So I hope there will be changes made in the building specifications of nursing homes over the next ten years.

Already, plans have been implemented in Canberra to build a new nursing home like the community-based village exclusively for Dementia patients in Holland and Sweden. The nursing home is set in a village scenario, including a shop, bus stop, and familiar things have proven helpful in these European nursing homes to people with Dementia.

As so many nursing home residents have died during the pandemic, it seems infection control processes need to be altered. Hopefully, future building regulations will allow for a separate wing for residents with a serious infection. This should enable complete separation of healthy residents from those who are seriously unwell. During the pandemic outbreak in some nursing homes this proved not to be possible, so the virus spread rapidly through the whole residence.

Implementing some of these suggestions and recommendations could save many lives in the future. Quality of life has to be considered in choosing a nursing home – but also keeping residents alive is of prime importance.

After Fulton died, I think I was suffering from post-traumatic shock. For so long, all my energy had focused on caring for Fulton and I had neglected my own health and wellbeing. I had experienced and seen things I would have thought impossible before my Dementia journey commenced.

Sharing my experience with Blanche helped me to heal and I hope writing about my journey will help other carers navigate through their own Dementia journey. The more I learned about the nature of Dementia along this journey, the lighter my burden became. Using the knowledge I gained has caused me to become an informal advocate for other carers. It has been their many questions about how to best care for a person with Dementia that led me to write this personal account in the hope it will help others navigate through their own carer pathway.

Know that as you commence your Dementia journey, you are not alone and reach out for the help that is available.

BLANCHE'S STORY

Dear Jenny
What positive insights!

I too feel the same with my new-gained informed perspective of Dementia caring. I hope to be the face-to-face connection that you provided me when I took on my novice caring role ...

***

You can never get to look back at the past or have hindsight until you have actually played a big role in a life-changing experience. This is exactly what Jenny and I did as carers to our husbands, who were both diagnosed with Dementia with Lewy Bodies, and who both lived with the Dementia symptoms for several years.

Now in hindsight, I wish to outline the final element of those choices made at the time – and how differently we would respond now.

We both learnt very early to remain focused with our carer's roles, to learn, to observe and to understand the meaning of Dementia a little better, to get over the significant hurdles that Dementia puts in your way. It is often not easy to decide or know how to act after an incident at short notice. With Dementia, one minute everything seems fine, and the next minute for no apparent reason everything changes and suddenly you find yourself in a pool of tears.

Yet slowly we learnt there is no other way out but to learn to accept and manage the stress and confusion that comes with the job of being a carer. To learn new ways needs time as Dementia alters one's life so drastically. That time becomes the main essence in the Dementia world: a carer needs time to adjust to the new norms, time to adapt, and considerable time to obtain the Dementia diagnosis. The important lesson here is to learn to forget the past – and to live in the present and explore future possibilities.

I am now aware that Dementia is extremely complicated to diagnose early. You have to go through a series of tests to achieve a correct diagnosis. By the time Jack's tests were complete, the Dementia signs were pretty clear, and damage to the brain was well under way.

One reason why Jack and I were so active to get an accurate early diagnosis, as we thought it would be best while Jack was still able to respond clearly to questions and express his concerns. Apart from the extra time we would have to plan, legally, financially and emotionally, for when Jacks's condition would decline further. Another important point to raise here is that Jack saw the need to participate actively in his treatments and trials whilst he was in control.

I now see clearly the efforts Jack and I made to chase for an early diagnosis were a waste of time. They were of little benefit, despite following all the right processes and instructions, to eliminate other medical possibilities that can be managed with the help of medication. Despite them, it took six years before a formal Dementia diagnosis was actually delivered!

Just as there is no cure for Dementia yet, nor is there a quick fix to halt the early signs of the disease from taking hold.

Looking back at our medical consultation, the doctors always stayed on focus to check for any underlying treatable conditions, like abnormal thyroid function, blood pressure or vitamin deficiency, as these disease can sometimes mimic cognitive difficulties and at no time was memory loss the focus of medical intervention.

Even though Jenny's and my Dementia journeys have run their full course, we are now using the present to reflect on the past choices we made when we were carers.

On the whole, I see some of the choices I made were real winners while others were simply bad. The important lesson to be learnt here is that learning can only happen by actively engaging.

Medical intervention just does not fall in one's lap, a carer has to go looking. The job of the medical profession is to hear you out, and for carers to spend time learning how to decipher the information that is delivered in a mosaic way. I had to learn to navigate the maze by being continually vigilant to handle a whole cascade of issues – and to confront the reality of the situation at the same time as living in a carer's world.

Jenny and I are still very much immersed with Dementia learning, so the stories we present collaboratively in this book will give future carers greater moments of joy in the final years together with less anxiety. To inspire others, we feel that now is the right time, whilst our caring role is fresh in our minds.

I also want to make sure this window of opportunity that has been created around the world, with Dementia numbers on the rise with baby boomers entering old age, will not close, and our book will be a guide. There is no other way out from this complicated, terminal and progressive illness, but to stay focused.

There are four main characters in our book, Jenny and me and our husbands. It is just not any dementia story, but it is our real lived stories. Some of the stories may put a smile on your face, others may bring about loud laughter, even though it was not at all funny when it played out. But the ending is sad because we do not get to live happily ever after.

Nonetheless, we are determined that our real lived stories compiled in a book will not be filed away like a research paper or academic journal. We struggled for so long and decided to write our book to help carers and health professionals to understand the carer's side of the disease.

I benefited enormously with the support I received from Jenny from the start to the end of my Dementia journey. A carer's life is traumatic, as the world you find yourself in is suddenly slipping. But another carer can feel and understand the pain and can connect more easily, because we share a common bond in Dementia care. I was blessed to be introduced to Jenny by a family friend and with Jenny's continuing support, the journey was made easier.

It would not be at all helpful to go it alone when the Dementia diagnosis is given. If for what ever reason a carer feels strongly they should shut out the outside world, it is important to ask, what is the reason behind the silence? Is it shame? Or stigma?

Shame and stigma exist, as Dementia is sometimes seen as a mental illness. But the only solution is to embrace the diagnosis and move forward with the support around you. Learning new ways to process grief slowly, talking to other carers in a supported environment, actually worked for me! Counselling, community support groups and Jenny's backing helped in my caring role. Importantly, none of these supporters painted a rosy picture of Dementia care. I would hate the thought of going it alone, by shutting the experience away and pretending that it is not happening.

In retrospect I would tackle my caring role very differently. I am a different person now, after my journey and so is my instant gut feeling. My carer's experience has given me the tools to see and evaluate certain choices that appear at different stages of the disease. They often played out differently in each episode and cannot be painted with the same brush. Dementia stages sometimes overlap as it is not necessarily linear, and caring only works if you learn to adjust and remain flexible to meet the needs as the disease evolves.

Being a novice carer, I struggled and found myself ignoring the early trigger symptoms of the emerging disease. I had more misunderstanding rather than a clear focus to understand the early symptoms. This was largely due to my ignorance. I faced fear when Jack displayed regular symptoms of his early impaired thinking, memory and communication loss, and I just brushed it off as an ageing process. I found it difficult to accept Jack's scattered thoughts, his self-conscious behaviour when we had visitors, when he over-thought every decision without being capable to make a firm decision.

This is another extreme example. But it serves as a good reminder that we all experience Dementia matters differently. The lightbulb moment switches on for carers at different stages. This is because we all bring different strengths, weaknesses, priorities and motivation in our caring duties. Understanding and accepting the disease varies for each of us.

In the early years Jack was relentless. He was determined to find a cure and he fully drove the process to get help to regulate his early memory behaviour, as he saw his constant memory failings totally undermining his confidence.

I fully supported his decisions to implement change. But on reflection, it was a lost battle. Subsequently, our world fell apart after several years of looking for an early medical intervention, when the Dementia diagnosis was delivered.

Although we expected it, nothing really prepares you. Jack chose to shut out the world momentarily, as he felt safe in a small world of his making and consumed himself with the injustice of the diagnosis. Especially as he actively implemented mitigating measures for several years, and felt severely let down by the medical profession. Psychologically, Jack became anxious, terrified, knowing he had an incurable degenerative disease that was going to rob him of his independence that he treasured as much as life itself!

With hindsight I would now let the disease run its multiple stages. Each stage brings its own characteristics, and gives the medical professionals a better picture when the Dementia symptoms are more obvious. That allows the team of medical experts to shape the treatment process.

Before the Dementia diagnosis was delivered, my journey began with raw emotions when everything in the world I had known and relied on was slowly shifting. Suddenly I found myself managing all tasks – both at home and outside. I had no one to talk about the finances. I had to contract services as I could not do it all. Searching for nursing homes became a clear priority soon after the diagnosis, as it requires time. Administrative paper piled up, with more forms to fill and file, so you know where to access them when required.

Besides having to cope with Jack's memory difficulties, the bigger concern was his personality changes that affected our relationship. Jack sometimes acted out and accused me of having an affair – it was no longer possible to have a logical conversation. Sometimes I felt I wanted to pack my bag and leave. Dementia statistics show this is often the case, either before or after the Dementia diagnosis. But most often couples stay put, because of the years of shared love – and accepting that it is not your partner speaking but the disease.

In time I accepted that the old Jack who loved to travel, who was energetic and enthusiastic about life, who made me feel safe when he was by my side, and who was easy to converse with, was gone. A stranger had now moved in and I could no longer depend on him to work together, despite him following me like a shadow!

Astonishingly, when I kept seeing Jack's peculiar behaviours, I knew he was not doing it to annoy me. Despite the inconclusive test results that we were handed for years, I knew that in essence living with a person with Dementia is just a matter of attitude, a matter of intentionality, and a matter of choices a carer makes to create a new normalcy.

My intention here is to inform and share the emotional impact the disease has over both the Dementia sufferer and the carer. Now, after the event, I have better insight to accept the issues surrounding this condition.

Comfort came to me by losing myself in other people's Dementia stories that I sourced through the internet, insightful blogs written both by Dementia sufferers and their carers. I found these well-written real lived stories, vivid and cathartic.

Community support groups were also a valuable asset in my journey, allowing me to create a rich internal world to counter-balance the outside complexities that I faced daily.

These activities made a big difference in alleviating my stress levels. With a clearer understanding of the disease, and by reading these stories, I knew I was not alone or hard done by with the Dementia diagnosis.

The real Dementia stories I sourced gave me the resilience to accept that Dementia is a progressive and an irreversible disease, that Jack's mind would not change or improve. In time the brain will essentially disappear when the disease takes a tight hold.

In recent times, both in Australia and worldwide, high profile celebrities with their families and community leaders are joining together in the fight against Dementia with their commitments to help raise awareness and to understand the disease by advocacy measures. This is indeed a welcome relief for families and carers. Along with films like *Still Alice* playing on the screens worldwide.

Jack would have hated his existence at the nursing home where he had to depend on others. I can hear him say, 'I am just existing and not living.'

Science at this point has still not figured a way to restore a person's memory and has a long way to go before a cure can be found, even though certain medications are known to slow the progression. But a lot more research needs to happen. Media news reports certain promising drugs. Though they can remove plaque from the brain, they are still clinically considered of little benefit.

Access to Dementia resources, treatments and even help to reduce the symptoms was only accessible to us after the diagnosis was made.

With little support in the early stages, carers have to muddle along. Doctors do not have enough time in a consulting timeslot to explain. We incurred steep financial costs, despite having Medicare and private health insurance. Medicare refunds are shamefully inadequate, especially the rebate you receive for a specialist visit.

The bigger issue here is the loss of our precious time together waiting in medical rooms, and then often leaving the surgeries none the wiser. In the early stages when Jack's symptoms were considered to be moderate. In retrospect, I wish I had not wasted those countless hours in doctor's waiting rooms, but rather had pursued a lifestyle that now would leave me with memories to cherish.

One incident that was extremely stressful. I decided to take a trip with Jack to Italy after his Dementia diagnosis. In hindsight I should not have travelled with Jack and now see it as plainly wrong. Jack's GP, the neurologist, the memory clinic and the family totally approved of our travel plans to holiday with our daughter in Tuscany and visit Jack's family in Holland.

Looking back, our decision to travel overseas was inadvisable. I would never recommend making travel plans with a Dementia patient, especially not a big trip to Europe. I now fully recognise my error – as the long flight played havoc with Jack's brain and he had a delusional attack when we landed at Milan airport. It took days to get Jack back into rhythm and even longer to get him to follow some sort of a routine, that in the end we abruptly cut our trip short.

Routine, consistency, planning and predictability is foremost for positive caring for any type of Dementia.

When I did my searches for a nursing home, including when I took the guided tour at the nursing home when Jack was offered a place, my Dementia knowledge and the idioms used were severely limiting, making it impossible to have any insight as how to frame the appropriate questions to get clear and useful answers. Unknowingly I put my focus on the visible structures of the nursing home, like the food on offer, and not sufficient focus on the care staff, to observe the way they interacted with the residents under their care.

Every institution has its own array of words and nursing homes are no different. A full lock-up facility, I learnt, meant the immediate nursing home surrounds allowed residents to move freely in a fully secure space, but residents were unable to get to the exit gate.

Yet Jack's admission is solely dependent on the ACAT assessment, and that is what decided that Jack would be placed into a low-care unit. A resident living in such a unit is still capable of living independently with limited care staff on duty at all times. They keep a watchful eye and occasionally provide help if the resident is having a bad day.

Make sure you have a lawyer or at least a second person to read the nursing home contract, before you sign the bond. I had an issue after Jack passed away to receive the bond refund.

I noticed a discrepancy and brought this error to the notice of the accountant of the head office of the nursing home, who admitted to the error and fixed it immediately. I had had no dealings with the head office. All administration was done at the nursing home for Jack's entry. However after Jack died, I found there was a complete break with his nursing home – and all queries were addressed to the head office.

I will forever feel traumatised when my thoughts take me to the day when Jack managed to escape from the nursing home to find his way home. At that stage, Jack was housed in a low-care unit, and managed to walk out in broad daylight, wandering aimlessly in the vicinity of the nursing home precinct for several hours, until he collapsed on the street from sheer exhaustion. A local school called an ambulance, and he was taken to the nearest hospital to the nursing home as he was unable to speak to give his personal details to the ambulance staff. Sadly, Jack's absence was not noticed at the nursing home until the nursing staff on duty received a phone call from the hospital, just before the evening meal.

The next day when I requested a meeting with the nurse manager of the nursing home, I was clearly made aware that the nursing home where I had placed Jack was not a full lock-up facility and it was not their responsibility.

I did not press the issue further although I was severely shaken with the response. I never expected a Dementia specialist to make such a remark, as she was aware that Dementia is shrouded in uncertain behaviour and most often difficult to get right, even for professional carers. Being my first and only complaint in the 12 months of Jack's stay, I felt there was no point in making waves, as Jack was safe and unaffected after the ordeal – and I was generally happy with all the staff and the level of care he received daily.

If I had to place a family member into a nursing home again, I would first check if the nursing facility was fully secure and what measures were in place to ensure that all residents are safe and unable to leave the building unsupervised.

The nursing home immediately increased safety measures after this incident, with Jack wearing a bracelet that would set off the alarms when he approached the exit and a roll call was taken each day, just before afternoon tea break.

The Dementia journey has also equipped me with clearer insight and foresight. Choices that seemed difficult in the past now seem clear, as I know how to approach choices that are available in the community. A carer has to have their eyes open. Nothing falls into one's lap.

As a result of my Dementia journey and experiences, I have now made a conscious effort to add certain health measures to my lifestyle. To maintain my overall health and to keep my brain active, I follow a healthy diet, drink plenty of water, engage socially, have arrangements in place for good brain exercises, read, learn a new language and importantly make exercise a vital part of my daily living. Research shows a healthy lifestyle builds cognitive reserves and helps to prevent the Dementia disease taking hold.

I have learnt new ways to adopt workable guidelines to accept the disease, with a more mature insight, that is required to stay mentally strong and to cope with the rollercoaster existence that runs several years. Even though I was disciplined, it is not always easy to stick to these guidelines with the constant interruption from caring duties.

Nor would I give unsolicited advice to someone going through the Dementia journey, not even if I had a somewhat similar experience in the past – unless my opinion was requested. I found it very annoying as a carer with different advice coming from all sides, especially from people without any Dementia experience or understanding. I know this can be difficult, as we all want to comfort the people we care for and let them know they are not alone.

Most annoying was when I got told, 'I know how you feel.' Though not intentional, it is really annoying hearing this comment, as these people have not had the experience of what it is to be a carer. The best advice is to just listen.

Both the Federal and NSW governments in 2020 saw an aged care crisis in nursing homes due to the Covid pandemic. In 2021, the Royal Commission into ageing made its report to bring better services and solutions, and to protect the basic rights for all individuals who live in aged-care facilities.

When Jack went into palliative care, I made sure he received care that radiated peace and comfort. I made sure he had his personal belongings, along with his music. I handed his end of life plan to the palliative care nurse. It goes into operation as soon as palliative care begins. Though, again anecdotally, it appears that some families have a greater problem because they are reluctant to face that their loved one is dying and so they do not want to decide on an end of life plan. This makes it difficult for the medical staff to know how to tailor the end, without any clear directive.

It was heart-warming to see the dedication of the palliative care team, and how much they do to make death comfortable. To a considerable extent it depends on the important document that is the end of life plan – and how we as his family tailored it to the values that Jack held. We had often discussed it casually, long before his Dementia began.

In 2020 and 2021, pandemic caring is an uncharted territory around the world, with services stretched to their limits and sometimes unable to offer supportive critical care to all those who need it.

For Dementia sufferers being cared for at home, it became even more difficult with total lock down. Most communities and care services closed for months. Carers had to do all their caring without any set routine and total breakdown of all care services to the home as well.

Dementia carers have to think ahead and make alternative plans for care management, in case the primary carer should become sick.

Jenny and Blanche's tips:
Hindsight-itis

- Keep a diary documenting your Dementia journey.
- Visit the person you have been caring for as often as possible, at different times of day or night.
- Lobby for improvements in nursing home care.
- Look after your own health.
- Reach out for support – for yourself.
- Don't be prejudiced by your preconceived ideas on what a nursing home should be. Visit them, speak to staff, residents and families and then make your own informed decision.
- To give good care, accept and understand Dementia.
- Accept the illness for what it is and do not chase a cure.
- Let go of any guilt or regrets from the past.
- Accept the Dementia journey is long and uncertain.
- Accept the long gap from the first symptoms to diagnosis.
- Learn ways to let go of the carer's role after the event.
- Address the carer's health when care duties come to an end.
- Move forward and focus on a wish list of things to do.
- Focus on personal growth.
- Stay focused to grow physically and mentally after Dementia.

Authors' note

Blanche and Jenny to this day appreciate that their friendship, although founded by their connections with Dementia, is no longer defined by their caring journeys.

Their lives are filled with laughter, life and love of family and friends.

We both wish you the best on your caring journey and hope our stories help you to navigate the road ahead – on your Dementia journey!

Carpe diem.

Acknowledgements

I was invited to write this book by Jenny Muir as we both struggled to understand the early symptoms of the Dementia illness, that evolved daily and differently for each of our husbands. I agreed with Jenny as I knew there was a large audience group who would benefit from our lived stories, as our research is our lived experiences, and in our writing we share our valuable insights, opinions and hindsight.

Our special thanks to Fiona Muir, who was instrumental in making sure we were on track and never gave up and made sure we didn't either. This is the reason the book has seen the light of day and she diligently edited our writing no matter how many rewrites it took. Thank you.

Special thanks to my children, whose support came readily when stressful situations occurred; my sister Jessie visiting Jack in my absence; and my many friends for their ongoing years of support.

Blanche Antonisen

I wish to acknowledge and thank all my children for their loving support during our Dementia journey.

My collaboration with Blanche on our joint narrative survived many detours and difficulties on our Dementia journey, not least of which was at times living on different continents and a number of Covid lockdowns. I am grateful we met by chance as carers for our husbands and that this first tenuous bond developed into a strong and lasting friendship.

Fiona provided invaluable support on many occasions when I was ready to give up. Her considerable computer expertise enabled me to overcome my own lack of computer literacy. At all times she maintained her equilibrium – even when I 'lost my manuscript somewhere in the cloud'. My manuscript would not have evolved into a book if not for her practical assistance and motivation to keep me going till I finished this journey. So thank you, Fiona.

I also wish to acknowledge our editor David Whitbread who has ensured our manuscript has finally been published, marking the end of our Dementia journey.

Jenny Muir

Made in the USA
Monee, IL
04 November 2026

67377019R00148